AGING BEYOND WELL

⎯⎯⎯⎯⎯⎯⎯⎯⎯⎯⎯⎯→

THE BIOHACKING SECRETS TO LIVE YOUNGER,
HEALTHIER, HAPPIER, SEXIER, LONGER ...

Ivel De Freitas, MD

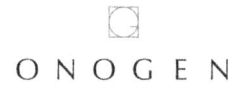

Copyright ©2022 by Ivel De Freitas, MD

Cover Photography: Elisa Stambouli

ebook ISBN: 979-8-9857936-4-2
Softcover ISBN: 979-8-9857936-5-9

No part of this work may be reproduced or photocopied without the prior written permission of the copyright holder and the publisher.

The information presented is the author's opinion and does not constitute any health or medical advice. The content of this book is for informational purposes only and is not intended to diagnose, treat, cure, or prevent any condition or disease.

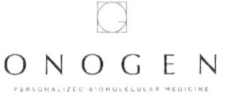

In Aging Beyond Well, Dr. Ivel De Freitas offers a ground-breaking paradigm shift on how we approach aging, with insights into new and promising pro-longevity and healing strategies aiming to help you become a healthier and happier version of yourself!

> —Mark Hyman, MD, Medical Director of the
> Cleveland Clinic Center for Functional Medicine,
> 14X New York Times bestselling author

I have been conducting research on the future of humanity for decades, including the topic of public health - a field dominated by technical progression and big pharma funding; a field characterized by dynamics that look promising and intriguing, but also: highly concerning. Who wants to live in a world where AI took over humanity, or where tech-companies decide what should be treated, and how? This book breathes fresh air and sanity into our medical future. The scenario sketched by Dr. De Freitas isn't naive, nor is it tech-averse. Instead, it brings about a world in which our health is being governed in a way that is holistic, empowering, integrative and preventive.

> —Dr. Roanne van Voorst, PhD, Futures-anthropologist,
> University of Amsterdam

In Aging Beyond Well we are introduced to the fascinating new biomedical field of biohacking. Dr. De Freitas guides us on an exploration of new ideas which tap into our body›s natural ability to heal and fight age-related disease. Aging Beyond Well is a penetrating and enlightening journey of discovery into a new era of medical advancements for anyone wishing to live and age well.

> —Ian A. White, MS., Ph.D, Founder and CSO, Neobiosis,
> Member of the Board of Directors,
> the American College of Regenerative Medicine

In Aging Beyond Well, Dr. De Freitas shares new, practical and easy strategies to help you improve your health and age well while bringing a refreshing insight and innovative ideas on how to support the shift of our current healthcare model towards a more advanced, participative, empathetic and inclusive healthcare system.

> —Juan Rivera, MD, Chief Medical Correspondent for the
> Univision and author; 2020 Top Health Influencer

I have known Dr. Ivel De Freitas for almost 10 years. I met her when she was the attending physician for my mother at Aventura Hospital in Florida. I noticed that when she showed up my mother's face always lit up. She was happy to see her. Other physicians were nice, professional, but did not bring a smile to her face. I also noticed that the residents and interns who followed her during her rounds were usually in good mood. Smiling, chatting, engaging with my mother. The whole energy of this little troop was warm and caring. That is why I stopped one evening as she was coming, and I was leaving. I thought, "This woman has a special energy, and she might appreciate my theoretical work on love." I told her that I worked with a new theory of love, and was she interested. She said yes. I sent her some information and we began a dialogue. I later found out that she had done a lot of studying other people's concepts about love – like Eva Selhub, MD, who wrote the Love Response, and others. She started to do what any good scientist would do, test the theory on herself. After a month or two of questions back and forth, she announced that in fact it made a difference in her life. That she was going to apply to her family and friends. After another month or two she was ready to test it on her patients. A couple of years later she asked me to be on her clinical trial team. That clinical trial at Danbury hospital lasted 1½ years, with the results being presented to the American Medical Association, where Michael Tutty, VP of Physician Satisfaction was extremely excited to hear our successful approach to preventing and alleviating the symptoms of physician burnout.

In short, Dr. Ivel de Freitas is truly a scientist who has been able to triumph over the medical establishment's reluctance and has integrated functional medicine with loving unconditionally into her approach to healing people. So glad she decided to write this groundbreaking book. Using science and her own transformative journey toward wellness as the framework and enriching its power with love, spirituality and poetry as her clarion call, this book promises to be life changing for many!

**—Stefan Deutsch, Psychotherapist, Author, and Founder of The Unconditional Life© Program,
President at Global Human Development, Inc, and
originator of new theories of love, aging and lifespan**

Dedication

For my patients and family!

Thank you for believing in me and supporting my forward-thinking ideas, honoring me with your trust and allowing me to use your stories to enrich the lives of others.

Contents

Dedication — v
Foreword — ix
Introduction — xiii

PART I: THE FOUNDATION

CHAPTER 1
Breaking Paradigms — 3

CHAPTER 2
Connecting the Dots — 25

CHAPTER 3
The Final Breakthrough — 47

CHAPTER 4
Genes Are Not Your Destiny — 81

CHAPTER 5
Telomeres, DNA, and Immunity: Turning Back Your Body Clock — 97

PART II: THE PROTOCOL

CHAPTER 6
PRIME — 117

CHAPTER 7
RESET   147

CHAPTER 8
GO   179

PART III: THE FUTURE

CHAPTER 9
A New Era Has Begun   193

CHAPTER 10
The Four Pillars of Future Medicine   209

CHAPTER 11
The Best Is Yet to Come   223

Index   239

Foreword

Dr. Ivel De Freitas is a healer and visionary leader in the field of regenerative medicine. She is kind, loving, compassionate and brilliant, but most importantly, she is *passionate* about transforming the lives of her patients so they experience greater health and longevity. She is a physician who aims for excellence, particularly in attaining the best quality of life and outcomes for all who consciously choose to collaborate with her on their health care journey. Her academic credentials are impressive and include attaining an M.D. from the Universidad Central de Venezuela, followed by an Internal Medicine Fellowship at Yale University. She has been trained in Mind-Body Medicine at Harvard Medical School's Benson-Henry Institute and Integrative Nutrition and Health Coaching from the Institute of Integrative Nutrition at the State University of New York. She has trained hundreds of medical students and has been a faculty member of multiple medical schools.

I was introduced to Dr. De Freitas in 2018 through a colleague who knew there would be a synergy between our experience in using precision medicine to target and treat disorders of the brain and body. As the former Director of Neuroimaging Research for the Amen Clinics, I have an expertise in leading clinical trials in a psychiatric setting, utilizing neuroimaging data as an adjunct to a thorough medical history, cognitive assessments, neuropsychiatric assessments and comprehensive lab work to target and treat complex psychiatric disorders. The patients who would visit our clinics came from over 155 countries around the globe and often had complex, comorbid psychiatric disorders. The Amen Clinics has the largest brain SPECT imaging database, with over 200,000 scans. Patients would often come to our clinic as a last resort offering a glimmer of hope to those searching for symptom relief. Having worked in this setting, I have profound compassion for those who live with chronic neurologic and psychiatric issues, and I appreciate those physicians who think about treating disease by addressing nutrient imbalances and embracing a holistic approach. This is what Dr. De Freitas embodies, and it's why I have such an appreciation and respect for her work. Upon meeting Dr. De Freitas, it was clear that we were aligned in our mission of optimizing patient care and providing solutions that are innovative yet non-invasive to the body as a first-line therapy approach to healing.

I gleaned a greater appreciation of Dr. De Freitas' ability to *reverse* biological age through a precision medicine approach based on an individual's biomolecular and genetic makeup when she presented her work at a Healthcare Future Conference in Portugal. She discussed patients' success stories in reversing *biological* and *immunity age,* and I was impressed with her results. Imagine having a biological age of 70 and an immune system age of 53. In an era of Covid-19, we have learned that maintaining our immune system is foundational to health, and Dr. De Freitas has a blueprint to guide you in attaining that goal. I soon realized that her strategy was taking the foundational principles of functional medicine, nutritional and IV therapies to a new level, implementing a revolutionary approach she created called *Prime-Reset-Go*, which focuses on optimizing your *biomolecular core.* For those reading this term for the first time, your biomolecular core refers to the trillions of biochemical processes, genes, micronutrients, and cofactors within your cells that determine how well you age. With a robust biomolecular core, you can navigate life with greater ease, less stress, greater cognitive and emotional flexibility, and a more harmonious connection from a mind-body-soul perspective.

In *Age Beyond Well,* Dr. Ivel De Freitas gives you insights from the traditional approaches used in mainstream medicine and integrates them with the expansive field of regenerative medicine, where the boundaries of the healing potential of our body are continually being redefined. We are now in an era where terms like biohacking, telomeres, chromosome age, stem cells, epigenetics, methylation, autophagy, cellular senescence and longevity diets are part of the nomenclature. People are no longer content with being healed from disease; they want to extend their health span and lifespan.

As a neurobiologist, I have always had an appreciation for optimal health originating at the cellular level. In *Age Beyond Well,* Dr. De Freitas goes into the detailed protocols necessary to regain optimal cellular health. You will find that this not only encompasses dietary and lifestyle shifts, which she details in Part II of the book, but that there is a unique functional medicine approach to fully restoring cellular health, which is at the heart of her program. Following her *Prime-Reset-Go* protocol will help treat chronic psychiatric or neurological conditions (which she illustrates with moving patient stories) and will also create the foundational support to attain optimized health for a lifetime.

Dr. De Freitas' goal is to reverse nutrient imbalances at the cellular level so that your biological age (which is influenced by your genetics, lifestyle, and nutritional choices) is lower than your chronological age. Having treated hundreds of patients at Onogen, Dr. De Freitas has discovered that most age-related problems are due to a reduction in the nutritional reserve of the biomolecular core.

If you want to live a life of greater health, vitality, and longevity, *Aging Beyond Well* is the book for you. It will help you become more conscientious about your daily habits and open your mind to a novel, non-invasive approach to supporting healthy aging. For those who require more personalized care to treat a chronic condition, I encourage you to work with her in person and experience the *Prime-Reset-Go* protocol at Onogen.

Kristen Willeumier, Ph.D.
Neuroscientist
Author of *Biohack Your Brain: How to Boost Cognitive Health, Performance & Power*

Introduction

We are entering a new era.

An era in which many facts we've long held true are turned upside down. At the outset of the twenty-first century, with the finalization of the human genome project, the discovery of telomeres (one of the keys to our age and vitality), and the newer-generation DNA biomarkers of aging (referred to as "epigenetic clocks") we've gained a transformational insight into aging. This new insight is disrupting not only the science of age management and healthy longevity, but also accelerating progress in other important fields, such as immunology, oncology, neurology, molecular biology, and regenerative medicine. Indeed, so much progress has been made in the field of aging that some experts believe we will soon be able to "cure" it.

But how long can we really live? How good can those years potentially be? And which of all those thousands of available options regarding age management are worthy of trying?

Although we are definitively living longer, on the quest of redefining aging and longevity, we now know that the collective longing is not really for more years but for better quality in those years. A life where aging may not mean losing vitality and functionality physically, mentally, and emotionally but maintaining or even gaining it.

It is imperative that all of us participate in this transformative change in healthcare and self-care.

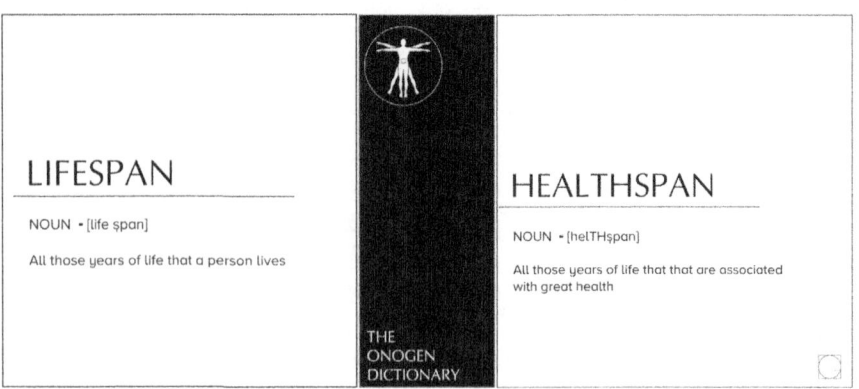

Living longer versus living better. Adding years of good health instead of just adding years to your life. Isn't this what everyone wants? Or perhaps a life that is not simply longer, but long enough for us to achieve feeling utterly perfect, happy, and fulfilled by becoming the absolute best expression of ourselves.

These are the secrets I'll be revealing for you throughout these pages. *Aging Beyond Well* brings a set of proactive practices and innovative therapeutics that I've learned throughout my personal journey as a functional, anti-aging, and regenerative medicine physician, as well as a daughter,

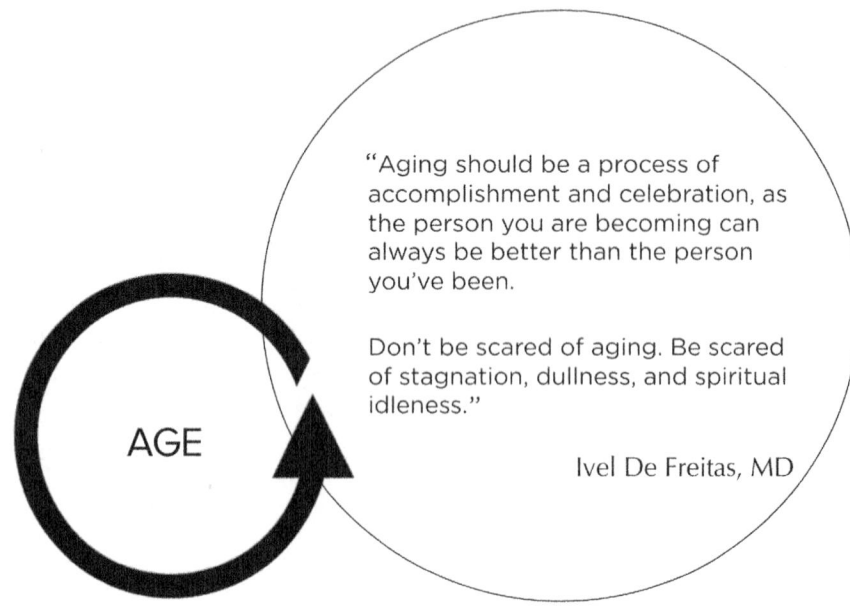

mom, and wife. With this, I hope I can help you shift your personal paradigm of aging, as I show you different ways to reset your biology and inner chemistry from stress and aging to healing, thriving, joy, and vitality.

The Biohacking Revolution

Mimicking the exponential pace of change in science and technology, the options available to us to meet our needs and pursue our goals are evolving rapidly.

The rise of the internet has also enabled most of us to access a broader spectrum of information and technology. At the same time, wellness tips, diets, health advice, therapeutic options, clinical trials, in-home testing, and hope are being constantly delivered to those who are either actively seeking or passively receiving health information on concepts such as human enhancement, extreme longevity, genetic blueprints, and precision and molecular medicine, which are now becoming topics of public and common knowledge. Patients are more empowered than ever to seek the most advanced care and are open to trying new biohacking options that

BIOHACKING

NOUN • [bīōhakiNG]

The activity of exploiting your genetic potential using the best of science and technology to achieve optimal health.

THE
ONOGEN
DICTIONARY

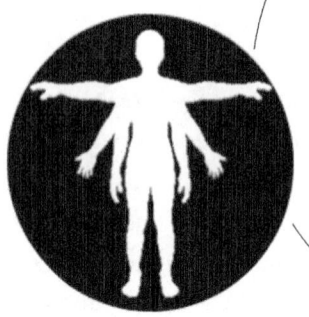

"Biohacking is not a trend, it is self-care 2.0, a shift in patients' mentality.

By embracing biohacking, we are literally supporting the shift of our current outdated medical model towards a more participative, equalitarian, empathic, and inclusive healthcare system."

Ivel De Freitas, MD

work with patients' own biology, their own genetic makeup, to achieve optimal health and well-being. Patients are no longer taking medical advice passively. They want to play an active role in their healthcare and medical decision processes. They want the latest and the best to be part of their medical plan.

People with this mindset are embracing a new empowering movement that is slowly but surely becoming a disruptive but positive revolution in healthcare: "The Biohacking Revolution."

Biohacking, understood as the use of technology and science to self-enhance health and well-being, is becoming the common denominator for modern self-care or self-advocacy—with new information, studies, and ideas being shared daily on the internet. Therefore, anyone with an interest in self-care who uses the internet—pretty much everyone today—becomes a biohacker, and biohacking becomes the new self-care.

It is imperative that all of us participate in this transformative change in healthcare and self-care—because it is for all our benefit. This new model understands that this rise of information availability makes us more empowered than ever, while it also makes us more vulnerable to scams, misinformation, and manipulation. This is one of the paradoxes of life in the twenty-first century: although the world changes rapidly and information is more available than ever, our basic needs as humans—love, empathy, identity, significance, contribution, connection—have not changed much. These human traits can be considered human strengths in most scenarios, but they can also make us vulnerable and can be used against us by scammers and those peddling false, unethical marketing.

The ideal model would deliver information freely but responsibly to educated users who understand how to navigate through this media-rich environment using critical thinking and recognizing red flags. For all of us, education and digital literacy are key.

Epigenetics: Understand the Potential of Your DNA

Along with this biohacking revolution, there is also an emergence of "new paradigms." The old assumption that your genes dictate your destiny is obsolete, as we now know that what is written on your blueprint is not nearly as important as what it causes your genes to express. In other words, though your genes may predispose you to certain conditions or diseases, for example, that does not mean you cannot impact your health and change your future.

Although it remains true that your DNA—your genetic code—provides the blueprint for your biological and molecular makeup, my work, combined with the work of many other researchers, points at your genes

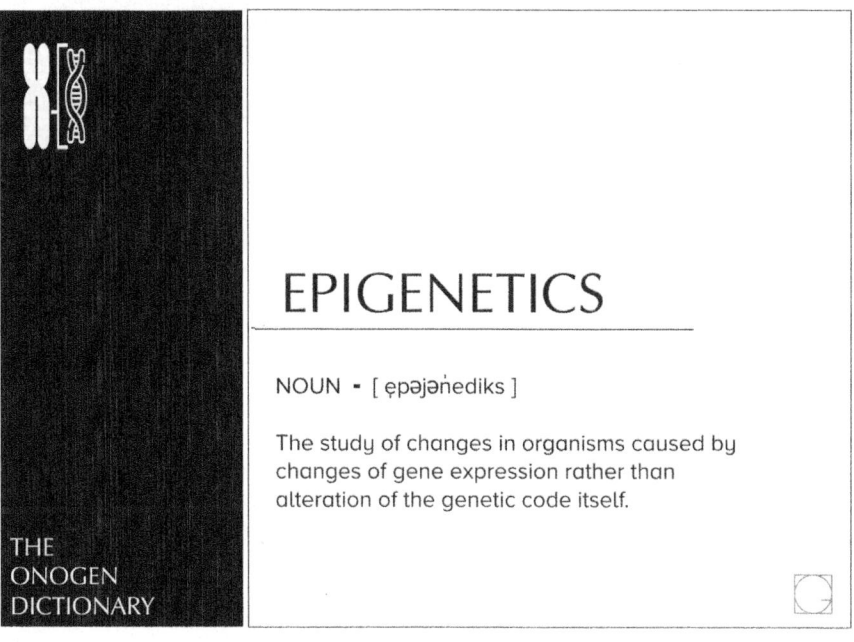

THE ONOGEN DICTIONARY

EPIGENETICS

NOUN - [ępəjənediks]

The study of changes in organisms caused by changes of gene expression rather than alteration of the genetic code itself.

as being more a prediction than a life sentence for you, which means that whatever is written in your genes will not necessarily happen to you. Indeed, some of your genes may not ever be expressed during your lifetime. Hence, why worry about a potential bad gene when you can channel your energy into learning how to keep those bad genes turned off? The "nature over nurture" paradigm has shifted to "nurture over nature" with the development of epigenetics.

Epigenetics has also opened the door to other new, empowering concepts, like biological versus chronological age and the "epigenetic clock," concepts that have emerged to prove you have more control over your health, well-being, physical/mental performance, aging, and longevity than you could ever imagine.

Recovering the Art of Medicine

Historically, medicine was founded on the concept of intuition. This concept, however, has been discriminated against and undervalued by the

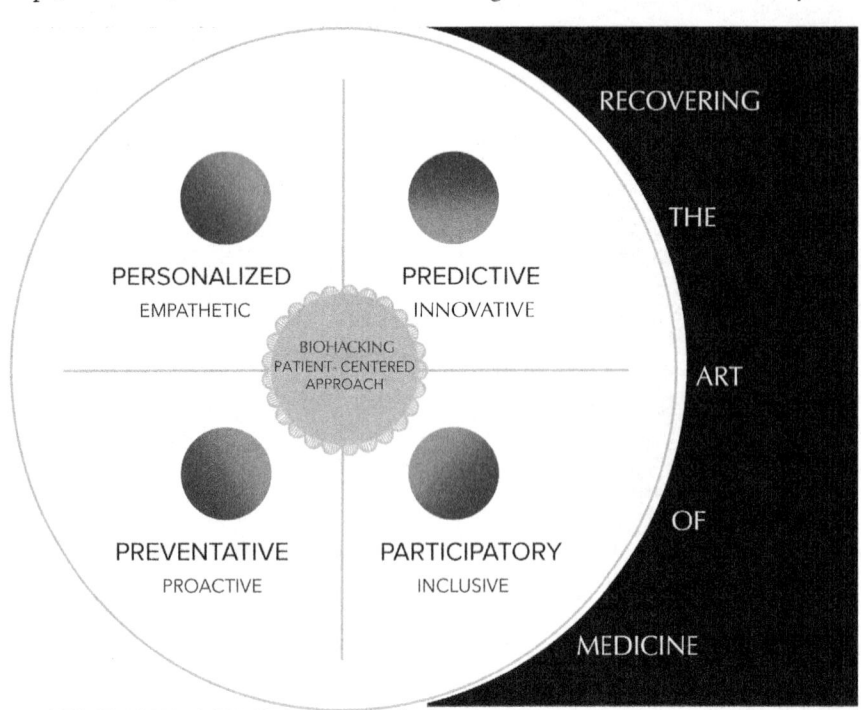

belief that medicine should be a factual science, where all decisions are made based on evidence.

However, despite medicine's absolute need for scientific discovery and standards, no one can deny the persistent presence and useful role intuition has in everyone's decision-making process. Albeit slowly, intuition, love, hope, belief, and faith are increasingly being recognized, based on an undeniable amount of evidence, as being instrumental for the care and healing of patients.

These concepts are the heart of the research and clinical practice I have proudly dedicated my life to and what moved me to create ONOGEN. As the founder of ONOGEN, my mission has been to set a new foundation for transforming healthcare and the existing medical model—a model that is failing to meet this new era of health literacy and biohacking. ONOGEN offers a model that helps us gather and interpret the increasing and at times overwhelming new data, while protecting physicians and patients from scams and manipulative marketing. My purpose in this book is to explain this new healthcare world and lessen the stress this information overload can cause.

I envision this new insight becoming a movement that champions patient preference, intuition, and values as equal to medical expertise, redefining the doctor-patient relationship and transforming and upgrading our healthcare model to a truly caring and loving one.

Is This Really Possible? Are We There Yet?

I want to ask you to take a few seconds to slow down, here and now. Perhaps you could even consider taking a few nice breaths.

I would love if you could help me to open your mind for just a few seconds and envision this:

Imagine living a life where just being well is no longer acceptable. Imagine stress is no longer an enemy but a mentor. Imagine yourself achieving your wildest dreams by unleashing your highest potential. Imagine that living a life of fulfillment is no longer an overused, unmet marketing promise; on the contrary, it becomes attainable to you and all human beings.

Imagine living a life where you wake up excited and full of passion and energy—like when you are in love or just achieved a major accomplishment in your life—and this becomes your status quo.

Imagine living a life where illness, ailments, and aging are optional.

Is this possible? Are we there yet?

The science, technology, and fount of knowledge available today have opened the possibility for you to accomplish many of these goals and even more.

We live in a time where most people are so busy and overwhelmed trying to survive in a constantly changing and demanding environment that there is almost no time to analyze and reflect deeply on complex data. Scientists conduct research, and most doctors just practice medicine, hardly keeping up with the overwhelming number of patients they need to see every day to sustain their practice. Thus, there is a natural gap between what is happening in the lab and what is happening in the medical office or in the hospital at the patients' bedside.

Inspired by this thinking process—and by my rebel habit of questioning and challenging the status quo—I decided to explore new and unpaved roads, translating complex scientific data into simple protocols that could be implemented safely into any patients' therapeutic plans.

As most of my ideas have developed and evolved throughout years of work with hundreds of patients, and the data on these novel strategies and

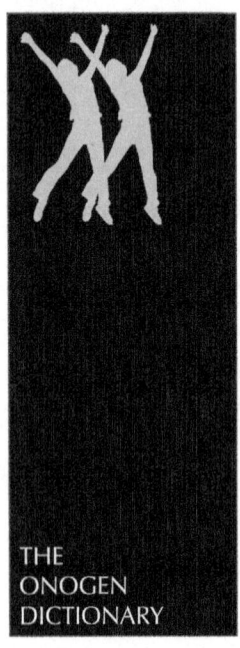

BEYOND WELL

NOUN • [bɪˈjɑnd wel]

Status of health and well-being where you live, operate, perform, look, and feel way beyond what you think "at your best" is. Allowing you to become the healthiest, happiest, and best version of yourself.

THE
ONOGEN
DICTIONARY

therapies is still developing, I have used my own patients' stories to illustrate the promising scope of these novel therapeutic strategies, combining it with the available evidence.

All the stories you will find documented in this book are authentic, but the patients' identities are masked to protect their confidentiality. Therefore, their names do not appear in the acknowledgments, but I still want them to know that I owe them a great deal for giving me the privilege to be their doctor, advocate, and friend, and for trusting and walking these unpaved roads with me.

My main hope is that by sharing these stories and the wisdom I have gained in the process, I can empower you with the knowledge and practical medical advice that have helped hundreds of my patients on this journey, helping you gain a deep understanding of the complex concepts that rule your health, well-being, and longevity, and helping you to find the path to biohack your healthspan. I hope I can inspire you to discover your unique personalized formula to live younger longer, empowering you to open the door to a new status of health and well-being that I have decided to call *beyond well*.

Going Beyond Well

This is a very exciting time to be a doctor as we are at an inflection point in medicine. We are witnessing a renaissance that will change the way we care for people. Concepts such as biohacking, precision medicine, nanotechnology, "one-size-does-not-fit-all," and even singularity and immortality are increasingly being discussed, researched, and utilized. Added to the technological blooming and advancement in artificial intelligence (AI), these elements are becoming the driving forces of this shift, which is pushing the current massive, reactive, and diagnosis-centered medical model toward a more personalized, proactive, and patient-centered model.

Although writing a book was on my bucket list, I had other things I thought that I needed to accomplish before doing so, in order to be ready for such a complicated and demanding task. However, life proved me wrong on this. While I kept ignoring the encouragement from my patients, colleagues, friends, and family, my ideas generated more and

GOING BEYOND WELL

NOUN • [ˈgəʊɪŋ bɪˈjɒnd wel]

Helping to bring the promise of elevated living, enhanced potential, and healthy longevity to all inhabitants of this planet.

THE ONOGEN DICTIONARY

more attention. Suddenly I found myself surrounded by colleagues and even hardcore scientists, functional medicine physicians, and biohacking, wellness, and bio-technology enthusiasts, who were interested in learning more about my work, ideas, and protocols. I could not believe it. In fact, at the beginning it was overwhelming for me. I was called names—the Alchemist, the Guru, and even the modern version of Ponce de León (one with a GPS, one of my patients said—that one really cracked me up). My therapies were called names too—the feel good therapy, the ultimate quick fix, the magic bullet, the elixir of youth... It became really intriguing to me how by just providing personalized and integrative nutritional and functional molecular support to my patients the outcome could be so positive and uplifting for them. I could not find any other approach in medicine that worked this way.

Was it possible that on my quest to find new ways to upgrade my patients' biology by filling the gaps in their biomolecular core I had come across a possible breakthrough in medicine? I kept asking myself: why me? However, the signs continued to intensify—until I had no other option than to accept the significance of my work and its potential implications and rise to the challenge to live up to all these new titles and the new

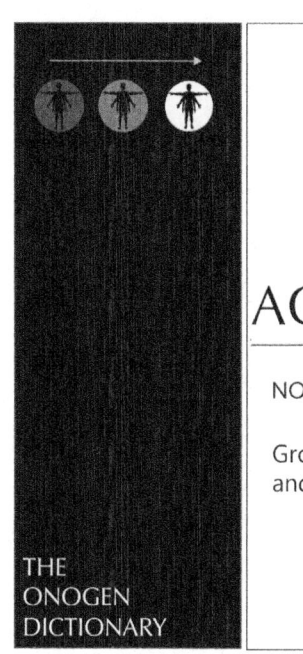

AGING BEYOND WELL

NOUN · [ˈeɪdʒ bɪˈjɑnd wel]

Growing and thriving into the healthiest, happiest, and absolute best version of yourself.

THE ONOGEN DICTIONARY

responsibilities that I'd been given. This implied that I had to give up playing small and get out of my comfort zone, to *Lean In* as Sheryl Sandberg describes in her inspiring book.

As my colleagues' interest increased, my confidence grew, and as I spoke up more, my path clarified. I understood better the power and potential of my work and, although still a "work in progress," it had already evolved to a point where I no longer could keep it to myself and for the benefit of just a few. As my fears started fading away, an urge to meet my responsibilities and share my work with the world prevailed. Therefore, I made the decision to write this book. It was clear! The world needed this information and was ready for it, so I had better be ready too.

In *Aging Beyond Well*, I encourage you to move your expectations in life forward, recognize your hidden potentials, and embrace living beyond well—a new status of health, where you enjoy a sense of elevated living, independent of your wealth, age, gender, or social status. A status where your body, mind, and soul display their highest potential, bringing into fruition new possibilities that may allow you to achieve way beyond what you have achieved up to now, accessing your unique talents, your superpowers.

SUPERPOWERS

NOUN • [ˌsuːpəpaʊə(r)]

A set of extraordinary abilities that any of us may potentially unfold, by aligning self-unique talents with purpose, discipline, and love, once self-biology has been upgraded. We all hold this mighty potential within.

THE ONOGEN DICTIONARY

Living and aging beyond well is you becoming capable of performing at the top of your game, at the absolute best expression of yourself in your everyday life. It is you performing in your superhuman mode.

Aging Beyond Well is me sharing my life story and my own awakening, growing, and healing process, reinforced by and intertwined with life challenges, lessons, and opportunities. A story that shares how I reshaped my practice, rekindled my passion for medicine and life, and juggled the journey with the responsibilities imposed by the multiple roles I was blessed to—a woman, a Latina, a mom, a wife, a daughter, a friend, a physician, a researcher, a dreamer, an entrepreneur, a CEO and Chief Biohacker... An adventurous, multi-passionate rebel—body, mind, and soul.

Aging Beyond Well is me dreaming big and hoping that my ideas could inspire others to join this initiative of redefining medicine and the healthcare system, initiating a process aiming to deliver more precise, proactive, empowering, patient-centered, personalized, empathetic, and loving care to be able to bring the very best out of each life we are honored to touch.

A transformed and transformational care system allows us to channel patients' intuition, instincts, and "biohacking" initiatives, instead of disregarding them. This, in turn, allows physicians and patients to team

Introduction | **xxv**

SUPERHUMAN

NOUN • [ˌsuːpəˈhjuːmən]

It's you, acting and enjoying life at your absolute highest biological, genetic, and emotional potential. It is you, once you have become the absolute best version of yourself.

THE
ONOGEN
DICTIONARY

up on the quest of helping each other become the absolute best version of themselves, redefining our roles for better, forever.

Call me an idealist. I know it is not easy to get to where my vision is directing me, but despite that, I recognize the process of incorporating most of these new concepts and practices into the healthcare system won't be quick and easy. A definite path forward is opening up, and I am excited to help push us in this direction, contributing to making this science available to all people.

Although, I humbly hope the information in these pages can contribute to the transformation of our healthcare system for the better. These words are mainly written for you, with the purpose of guiding you to craft a personalized practical and doable "biohacking" plan to achieve the *beyond well* status you deserve, taking better control of your health and aging process while becoming the highest, truest expression of yourself in your lifetime.

My hope is that you'll find this book life-changing and revolutionary, opening a new perspective on what you can accomplish in terms of your health and performance, not only for you, but also for your loved ones and every soul that your life touches.

I'm also asking you to please share and help me to get this message and science out in the world. Just imagine the potential this could have and the positive revolution this could start, if only we could unlock the potential of every individual in society, so they could perform much better. Wow! This would be a human enhancement project, where people could be healthier, more productive, more creative, happier, kinder, and more open-minded just by optimizing their biomolecular harmony and micronutrient environment. Imagine what our society could become!

Now, let's get this journey started. I just need you to keep reading and stay open-minded! Allow yourself to connect with your core, your real needs, your wisdom, your intuition. Perhaps, you might find, as I did, that this is just the perfect time for you to start a transformation journey!

Welcome Transformation!

Where to start to be able to transform our health and reality is a question I have been asking myself since medical school. Earlier in my career I learned that health was not only defined by the body's biology, but also by the mind and even by the environment. Hence, I understood that my job as a physician was way beyond helping the body to work better; it included guiding my patients to find their way through their life process. For some of them, this was a challenging journey bringing about profound changes that allowed them to emerge as a new persona. A persona that was more connected with their own needs but also with the needs of their loved ones and their environment. A process that many times revealed unknown talents and gifts.

In my personal process, I have discovered an unknown talent for writing poetry. Don't take me wrong, I always loved poetry, but I never knew I could write poems myself. Until one day after my morning meditation, while I was journaling, my ideas started flowing in rhyme. One of those days, I wrote the piece I am sharing with you here. A piece that became a personal proof of my awakening and growing. An inspiration and a reminder of the kind of world and healthcare system I wanted to be part of. The kind of world I wanted to collaborate on to build, for my patients, for my family, and especially for my children. A more loving, caring, compassionate, inclusive, embracing, participative, and egalitarian world—with a more loving, caring, compassionate, participative, egalitarian, and inclusive healthcare system.

Welcome to Our New World!

Today I wake up in a new dimension,
where possessions and armors no longer exist.
Where what you wear,
does not define you,
your mistakes don't leave any marks, and
"what you have" is not considered an expression of "who you are."

Where only our souls matter.
Where connections happen beyond words, agreements, and actions.
Where personalities, traits, agendas and purposes move to a second level.
Where motives and reactions are not more than circumstances,
and to forgive and be forgiven is no longer needed.

A truly new dimension,
where norms, rules, and traditions that govern us have expired, and
the status quo is already obsolete.
What is so much formality for?

After all, in this space the different points of views
—no matter how odd they are—
are now more than welcome;
being embraced and celebrated like
new colors added to the rainbow or
new notes coming into an already monotone musical space.

In this space...
love, gratitude, and unconditional support
become the universal language and currency,
while payments, coins, and invoices become meaningless,
they no longer fit.
In this space...
Feeling is more important than thinking.
Loving is more important than winning.
Helping is more important than trading.

In this space...
You can live and breathe peace.
Finally, discovering what "truly live" means,
embracing all of them who want to come in.
Feel welcome if you dare to check in.

Ivel De Freitas, MD

PART I

THE FOUNDATION

CHAPTER 1

Breaking Paradigms

If I ask you how you are doing, would you say you are doing well? How many times have you felt unwell, and doctors have told you that everything looks good and that by reviewing your labs, they can assure you that you are doing well?

"Well" is defined as a good or "satisfactory" condition of existence. Satisfactory? Really? How does this sound to you? Satisfactory equals sufficient, adequate, reasonable, average. Average? Really? *Is this how you want to be doing?*

I grew up in a family where the proper answer to the question of "how are you doing?" was: "I'm doing better every day." This is how my Dad used to and still answers every time he is asked how he is doing. Being just well has not suited me ever and sounds to me kind of like "not good enough."

Certainly, sufficient, standard, satisfactory, and average are not the way I want to be doing or I want my patients or loved ones to be doing, especially because I know now—and I have my amazing patients to prove it—that we all have the potential to live and feel way above and beyond those standards that we have accepted for many years as our status quo.

4 | Aging Beyond Well

STATUS QUO

NOUN • [stādəs ˈkwō]

The way things are now, a resistant state of existence, or in other words the traditional way of doing things that can always potentially be disrupted.

Questioning the Status Quo

What if I tell you, based on my personal and professional experience, that most likely you're operating, most of your days, somewhere below your highest potential and that no matter how successful you are, how good you feel, or what your physician has told you on your last check-up, you could be feeling and performing way better than what has become the standard for you. What would you say? How does this sound to you?

We all know there is always room for improvement. If you think and analyze carefully, you'll identify areas where you would be more than happy to see improvement happening. Perhaps your energy could be better, your brain could be sharper, your mood could be happier, your attitude could be more positive, your skin could be tighter and more glowing, or even your sex life could be spiced up and more erotically fulfilling.

We blame stress, aging, poor diet, sugar, environmental toxins, too much coffee, too little coffee, lack of sleep, bad relationships, poor digestion, difficult days at work, the modern lifestyle, lack of time, lack of purpose, poor health, poor self-esteem, depression, anxiety, and so on…. Thanks to *Aging Beyond Well*, we have no more excuses.

Stress is expensive! Well, not only stress, but also its triggers, in the form of modern lifestyle, environmental toxins, heavy metals, relationship strains, aging processes, and genetic mismatches that cost our biomolecular core tons of nutrients and essential biochemical factors. This means that stress impacts on your body wearing away your cellular micronutrient and biomolecular reserves, messing up your biomolecular harmony, by slowing down some of the trillions of biochemical processes occurring in what I decided to call your *biomolecular core*.

As your core muscles are the mechanical base of support for your entire body, your biomolecular core is the biomolecular base of support for your entire being, body, mind, and—based on my observations—I would dare to say your soul as well. Therefore, just as a healthy muscle core is essential to keep your body healthy and balanced, a healthy biomolecular core is essential to keep your body, mind, and even soul in good shape.

So while you are sitting or lying right there reading this book, and everything seems to be restful or still in your body, there are trillions of biochemical reactions happening at the same time in your biomolecular core that allow your mind to focus, your muscles to be still, and your soul to be connected with the current moment.

THE ONOGEN DICTIONARY

BIOMOLECULAR CORE

NOUN • [bai·aa·muh·leh·kyuh·lr kɔː(r)]

The trillions of biochemical processes, genes, micronutrients and essential cofactors within your cells that determine how fast you age, how good you look, act and feel and how long you live, by modulating your gene expression and tissue healing and regeneration.

You might consider this like an image on a computer or smartphone: what seems to be just a simple image on the screen is, in fact, a reflection of very complex processes happening on the inside, in its processor core. In the same way, the reactions happening in your inside, in your biomolecular core, allow your body, mind, and even your soul, not only to -do what you need or want to do every single moment, but also its balance is key for you to thrive and evolve in any of those areas of your well-being.

Your biomolecular core is working even while you are sleeping and meditating, and its lack of harmony or imbalances can translate into difficulty with these activities. Poor sleep compromises immune system function, natural healing, and recovery processes essential to keeping you healthy and performing at your best. Treating lack of sleep with sleeping pills instead of addressing the biomolecular source is not helpful to your well-being in the long run.

Just as the processor core and its processor harmony are essential for the optimal function and lifespan of your device, your biomolecular core's harmony is essential for your body and mind's optimal function and lifespan.

This means that a harmonic, well-balanced, and optimally functioning biomolecular core is not only crucial for you to display and enjoy optimal energy levels, mood, brain clarity, skin health and beauty, weight and metabolism, sleep, stress management, and even your libido, sex drive, lifespan, and healthspan, but also your spirituality, joy, peace, and serenity.

The depletion, imbalance, and dysfunction of your biomolecular core and reserves seem to explain, based on my clinical experience, the dramatic impact that stress has on the way your genes express and work. It also impacts your mood and how your cells, including the neurons in your brain, perform, recover, repair, and heal every day. In other words, stress causes a cellular supply-demand mismatch that ultimately impacts not only your performance on a daily basis but also your pace of aging and your chances of developing an age-related condition, such as dementia, cancer, heart disease, arthritis, autoimmune conditions, and immunosenescence—the decline of immunity—in the long term.

Contrary to popular belief, biomolecular reserves of fat-soluble vitamins, such as A, D, E, and K, and even some water-soluble vitamins like B12 and folic acid, have been documented in the body's liver and muscles. However, ideally the body should be replenished with most of them every few days for optimal cellular function. This is even more important when the body is under stress as the reserve are not usually enough to sustain optimal cellular function under these circumstances.

This means that when you are under stress, your cells need more than what you can provide by simply eating well, taking supplements, and trusting your reserves. I have seen this not only in patients following a poor diet and taking no supplements, but even those mindful and disciplined individuals who follow a wise and healthy diet and supplement regimen.

If you ignore, like I used to and most traditionally trained physicians do, what your unique and personal biomolecular core needs are, chances are you are not fueling yourself correctly, and eventually your warehouse or core reserve starts running down. This can negatively, slowly, and progressively impact your daily physical and mental performance, as well as your own capacity to deal with stress and repair and maintain your body! This creates biomolecular imbalances that compromise your recovery mechanism, and prevent you from enjoying deep sleep, a positive and happy mood, brain clarity, optimal energy, and the great sex life that you deserve.

Therefore, the best formula to live younger longer has a lot to do with the balance of your biomolecular core, and those essential missing pieces, your biomolecular gaps, that you require to keep your body working the way it is meant to work.

Understanding what your core is missing and formulating a personalized and comprehensive therapeutic plan to fix it should become a standard practice in medicine. However, the path we are on has been determined by pharmaceutical and health insurance corporations. Therefore, healthcare has been forced to sacrifice quality for cost, leaving many useful tools by the wayside in the hunt for financial sustainability.

Emerging from the COVID-19 Pandemic

The pandemic has come to challenge the status quo, transforming the way we live, work, and relate with each other, disrupting politics, economics, science, and education. It has also dramatically changed our perceptions of healthcare and how it should be delivered, bringing us a new insight to the key role nutrition plays in immunity and its capacity to respond and protect us against infections.

Immune resilience, is a new term use to define the ideal and balanced immune response needed to overcome COVID-19 successfully, as maintaining a balanced immune response is key to preventing respiratory failure and death caused by an exaggerated inflammatory response and the cytokine storm. Immune resilience allows the body to fight the infection, attacking and eliminating unwanted viruses, while still preserving the capacity to modulate inflammation, avoiding hurting your own body organs and cells during the process. For some people, this happens naturally, for others it doesn't.

It is now well-recognized that although a robust immune response is helpful at the beginning of an infection, lack of balance in such response can bring the patient to an unwanted hyper-inflammatory state that can lead to acute respiratory distress syndrome (ARDS), respiratory failure, multiple organ failure, and death.

Stress and aging-related chronic disease have both been linked to increased inflammation and poor outcome. We now understand that the link between aging and decreased immune response appears to be related to increased baseline low chronic inflammation, called inflammaging, and the deterioration of the immune response known as immunosenescence.

Immune resiliency depends on many factors including age, lifestyle, level of stress, nutrition, and health status. Many important lessons were learned during the pandemic, and I think one of them is not to take our immune system for granted. A rise of awareness on the importance of nutrition for optimal immune function has explained the increasing number of people taking vitamin C, vitamin D, and zinc.

While this is demonstrating some level of collective awakening towards this subject, nutrients have not been part of what the healthcare industry has included as standards of care in the management of patients admitted to the hospital with COVID.

The lack of attention and resources dedicated to fostering growth and development in these key areas explains why mainstream nutritional testing is still in a primitive stage, using only blood levels, which are static values that are pretty much inaccurate when trying to take a more proactive instead of the more traditional reactive approach to medicine. Therefore, some of your biomolecular needs are not being addressed at your annual doctor's appointment with its regular blood work and testing.

While cutting-edge functional genetic testing is still considered experimental by mainstream medicine. The general public is increasingly more open to in-home testing bought online and ordered by the end consumer without the need of a prescription for it. However, not all the information is out there yet, and there is much that is still in development, like the concepts I am presenting to you. Concepts that, in my experience, if you ignore—like I used to and most traditionally trained physicians do— might be compromising your health and daily performance in ways that you might not perceive initially.

First, even if you think you are the healthiest person on Earth—you take twenty supplements a day, your friends call you a "wellness freak," and you have spent years reading and educating yourself on diet, vitamin supplementation, and lifestyle—you are most likely still not meeting your unique biomolecular needs in some areas. You still have room to feel and perform better. You most likely are aging faster than you should and not feeling as great as you could.

Growing up in a family of entrepreneurs, one of the most common topics of dinnertime conversation was how to improve what we are doing right now.... How to make it better for us and for the company and the people in the company. For my parents, business was not just about profits, but everything from education to the health of the people who worked with them. I remember my parents talking about how to help this person to eat healthier and how to help this other one to get more inspired to go back to school. Their employees' potential was a normal topic for our family dinner. Helping others achieve their highest potential was one of the main goals I perceived my parents to have not only in my life but in the lives of anyone they touched. Everyone and everything can improve! That seemed to be my parents' motto, not only as entrepreneurs but also as mentors. and, of course, as parents. I am sure that this holistic, conscious, entrepreneurial focus during our upbringing had a lasting impact on me.

So, helping people and the premise "Why settle for good enough, when there is always room for improvement?" became the most important and defining lessons of my childhood.

Fortunately for my sister and me, this conscious approach to business was also applicable to parenting, so I have to say we were blessed by amazing parents and their love and guidance. This means our parents managed to balance love and discipline, and they applied this basic approach of loving discipline to every area of our life, our nutrition, health, and wellness included.

Being healthy at my home was pretty much one of our duties, so eating your greens and exercising were as important as studying hard and getting good grades. While we were always expected to deliver our best at school, our wellness and health were not excluded from this loving disciplinary approach.

We were so into wellness as a family that we started the weekdays with a family jogging session at the park at five A.M. I know it may sound kind of military for you, or even harsh, and what I am going to say might surprise you. I enjoyed jogging those mornings with my family. I realized at a very early stage of my life that this was a great strategy to help me manage stress and keep me focused and positive. So, this is how exercise became a part of who I am today.

As an eager reader, my interests were also almost exclusively health, wellness, and fitness. *Atkins, Pritikin,* and *Fit for Life* all went through my hands. Moved by the amazing health and well-being benefits described by the Diamonds in their book, *Fit for Life*, at the age of sixteen, I became a strict vegan and increased my fasting time by skipping breakfast. I am talking about almost thirty years ago, when this science was just in the hands of pioneers and paradigm breakers, and vegan and intermittent fasting were not a cool thing to do but on the contrary a crazy and challenging thing to do. My mom thought I had become anorexic or some similar disorder. Poor thing, I cannot imagine how concerned she was when she saw me losing all that weight and still stubbornly and rebelliously sticking to my original plan of not breaking my new vegan lifestyle. I guess this is part of the liabilities of raising kids who are eager to break rules and paradigms—that is how I was and still am.

In those days, I also raised my fitness goals and started training for competitive aerobics, so it was not a surprise that I soon became the diet and fitness guru of my school. I was involved in school wellness and fitness fairs, as well as in charge of the nutritional and fitness plan of many of my friends—without knowing at that time that this initial consulting and coaching at lunch was just the beginning and that I was paving the path to the rest of my professional life.

This is how I found out I wanted to be a doctor—but not a traditional one. I wanted to help my patients regain health through nutrition and exercise, just as I had learned from the books I'd been reading. I wanted to help break paradigms and to change medicine as those writers were trying to do. I also fell in love with the idea of helping people feel better just as I had in my short, informal health-coaching experience during school lunches and breaks. However, I embarked on this journey without knowing the challenges I would encounter in a very rigid space: medical school and academia.

I did not know then that there was not much room in medical school for my curiosity and open-mindedness. I did not know that in medical school "well" was good enough and that I would spend my next ten years so distracted and fascinated by the complexity of human anatomy, biochemistry, physiology, pathology, and pharmacology that the main reason I wanted to become a doctor in the first place would be washed out of me. So, by the end of medical school, I had mastered what by then I thought of as the art of medicine.

My fascination with the possibility of saving a threatened life with a pharmacological or medical intervention was at its highest level. I was in love with the path I had chosen, and I did not then question the methods. I was like a sponge. I absorbed as much as I could and proudly became another one of the providers of the "well is good enough" approach, and in this process, I also became tough, harsh, rigid, and arrogant!

Don't You Dare

Oh Lord! I was tough. In fact, I was terrible. I was the one who was assigned the troublemaker students or new residents in order to "fix" them. The good ones loved me and admired me, but the troublemakers felt threatened and intimidated by the idea of having to work under my supervision. My patients liked me, as I was always polite, kind, and empathetic, but I did not tolerate mistakes or laziness on my side. This was probably the main reason why I was loved by my attending physicians and used as a role model. Chief resident, preceptor, attending of the year were awards and responsibilities that were assigned to me throughout my educational path. I did not then question anything from academia and hardcore science.

Now that I think about it, I actually did a few times but not consistently enough to wake me up.

Here's a great example.

While doing my first residency in internal medicine in Venezuela, we used to get patients with tuberculosis occasionally. Tuberculosis, or TB, is a bacterial infection that usually does not make you sick unless your immune system is compromised. We mostly see it today in patients with severe malnourishment and AIDS in underdeveloped countries. I questioned once in a teaching round why we did not give these patients vitamins. It was obvious to me that these patients needed nutrients. However, the answer was that vitamins could decrease the effectiveness of the drugs and feed the bug causing the disease.

This is the same argument that traditional oncologists give me today every time I create formulas for patients in chemotherapy. For TB treatment, that argument has been proven wrong. In fact, these patients are now supplemented with vitamins as part of the standard protocol, mainly because there are studies that support supplements to prevent some of the worst of TB drugs' side effects.

One of the main culprits in the disease is the failure to nourish the body, resulting in a depressed immune system. Studies have demonstrated that incorporating specific nutrients into these protocols not only improves patients' tolerance to the TB drugs but also might help them rebuild their immune system and get better faster. But I challenge you to ask a doctor what the benefits of using supplements are while being treated for TB. The answer would be to prevent the drugs' side effects.

I hope that we can soon change this paradigm and create more awareness within the conventional medical establishment, and especially those from the infectious disease and oncology community, that nourishing and supporting the body's natural healing processes with the right nutrients and peptides is as important as choosing the right antibiotics and chemotherapy.

I really think that this is when ONOGEN was born as a concept. For sure, these early kinds of revolutionary thoughts and ideas became my inspiration later in life, and during the COVID-19 pandemic, I created one of our most successful therapeutics, our IMMUNITY GO Therapeutic Protocol.

IMMUNITY GO

NOUN - [iˈmyo͞onədē gō]

The therapeutic priming of your biology with micronutrients and peptides to boost your immune system during challenging times.

THE ONOGEN DICTIONARY

Looking back at my own experience first as a medical student and later as a faculty member of multiple medical schools, I realized the current educational model is not set up to foster free thinking, exploration, and questioning of the status quo—important concepts that have led to the innovation boom we have seen in other fields. While the world is witnessing an unprecedented technological boom, it seems to be missing medicine. In no other scientific field is change and technology received with so much resistance and skepticism than in medicine.

Of course, respect for tradition and routine in our field is paramount to mitigate risk in a profession centered on life and death. However, challenging the status quo should be an expected part of any thriving scientific culture—and medicine should not be exempt!

I know from my own experience that it takes more than courage to deviate from the paved path. To create a route to innovation, it is necessary to let go of the "way things are" first and welcome "the way they could be" and manage the uncertainty that this approach brings. Finding ways to encourage this mentality to embrace change is the key to fostering innovation. However, this requires a lot of flexibility and a sense of humility that is sometimes hard to find in our field—especially in our medical school leaders, where a simplistic culture of rank seems to be the dynamic of our daily lab practice and hospital medical rounds.

While in every other field innovation is being ignited by the youngest and most inquisitive minds, the strict medical hierarchy and the demanding and exhausting academic curriculum leave no room for free thinking and creativity necessary for these young minds to explore new ideas and propose new methods of solving challenging issues.

Guidelines, best practices, standards of care, medical associations and boards, insurance companies, Medicare, and the FDA are all meant to keep the field regulated and safe. But it is our responsibility as providers to keep challenging the system and to not miss opportunities to bring up ideas that could improve care and ignite innovation. This mindset needs to be fostered within academia.

Innovation should be wired into the brains of doctors and healthcare providers as much as it is in all technology careers. We need to carefully, kindly, and lovingly open space for innovation and development within our own medical curriculum and daily practice. System and practice improvement need to be at the core of our daily rounds, and creativity and discovery should be happening beyond the lab walls, at the bedside.

We all need to cooperate if we want to see more positive changes happening in our medical arena; after all, we are all part of it, doctors, providers, and patients alike. Innovation is ignited by necessity, and medical necessities are experienced in the field every day by each one of us. The missed opportunities start when we don't see them as an area of opportunity but as an unsolvable limitation. I think this is the disconnect we have between technological development and medical practice. Regulators and academia need to find new ways to allow innovation and creativity to become new key players in medical rounds, fostering more free thinking and exploration in the medical curriculum.

Creating a more open space for innovation and change within the medical arena is how we are going to start seeing more meaningful innovation in our medical practices and patient care. But the change has to start within ourselves, providers and patients alike, by taking individual responsibility and embracing change and innovation in a safe and positive way.

We need to change to a culture that embraces new technologies and ideas making it easier to be creative and open to serendipitous advances.

Innovation in technology, beyond electronic medical records and patient portals, is highly needed. Technology that would allow us to translate complex genetic and biomolecular data to create personalized protocols for each patient based on their unique medical, biomolecular, and genetic profiling. This is the quest that inspires me and my team to translate our research protocol results into algorithms, envisioning the ability to create an intelligent engine capable of delivering personalized wellness optimization plans specifically designed based on patients' unique biomolecular and genetic profiling to upgrade their biology and optimize their wellness, immunity, and overall healing capacities throughout their life.

The Wake-Up Calls

I had many wake-up calls throughout my life. Some of them were soft awakenings, where the universe was just whispering to me, but others came in the form of real crises. The first hit me during the earliest years of medical school .

I happened to be so fascinated with understanding how the body works and how healing can be triggered by different interventions that I disconnected from my own needs in the process. Skipping meals, late nights, tons of coffee, and very little sleep became part of my new lifestyle.

By the second year, I had my first health crisis: fever, fatigue, elevated liver enzymes with a final diagnosis of mono—also known as infectious mononucleosis or the kissing disease. I was a nineteen-year-old single girl back then. I did not know that making out could impart this risk! LOL.

My serology came back positive for acute EBV (Epstein-Barr Virus). For those who don't know, EBV has been linked to chronic fatigue and even increases your risk for some kinds of cancer. It took me a few months to recover completely. I couldn't run without getting a sharp pain in my abdomen in the upper-right quadrant—over the liver area. I felt exhausted. My brain was foggy. I was depressed. I could not find the joy, the energy, or the enthusiasm I needed to cope with my demanding lifestyle.

It took me six months to start feeling a little better. But it took me longer to get back to what I thought was my baseline. So, I adjusted and felt blessed that I could finally run again. I was not as fast and not as good, but who cared as long as I was running? I also started gaining weight for no reason. Weight that I would not lose for the next three years. At that time, I did not put it together, but I know now—my biomolecular core was struck hard, and my adrenals and metabolism were messed up because of it. My energy was not the same for a long time. It was after many years of being "good enough" with normal labs and standard energy that I discovered what my deficiencies were, how to replenish them, and what my real genetic potential was! I finally discovered my personal *beyond well* formula.

However, three years after my EBV diagnosis, before I discovered *beyond well*, I made it to my clinical clerkships. I thought I was doing well. I had recovered most of my energy—at least I thought I had—and I was working with patients, which had always been my dream. I started working nights at the Red Cross as a volunteer to increase my clinical experience, which was very demanding as my studying already compromised my sleep.

If you add my hospital volunteer work at night and the amount of stress with the clinical clerkship, my second health crisis should have been no surprise.

It was during my pediatric rotation when another crisis hit me. This time it was chickenpox. I was in my twenties and had a history of childhood asthma. My chicken pox rash and fever were complicated by difficulty breathing from severe pneumonitis, which meant my lungs were as infected and inflamed as my skin was.

This almost put me in the hospital, which would have forced me to lose many hours and credits that were vital for me to graduate with honors, which was extremely important to me back then. This added an extra amount of stress and drama that I did not need. Luckily, my system was resilient enough to get better quickly, and I found the motivation to pull myself together. I ended up overlapping two rotations and still made it through graduation on time and with honors, but with a lower GPA than I wanted.

I began to recognize a pattern that later I'd confirm. I recognized the toll my body was taking due to stress and the resultant unrecognized drop of my immune system. This motivated me to start questioning the current medical model, lab technology, and the status quo.

My health crises were all triggered by what seemed like well-managed chronic stress with a sudden spike that threw everything apart, like the last drop that overflowed the cup. A pattern that I slowly realized was also

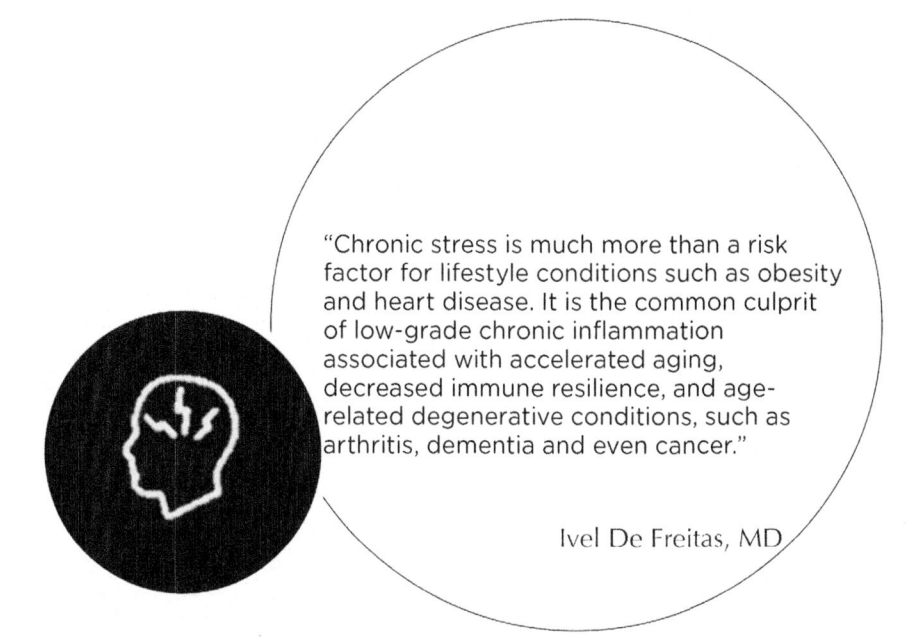

> "Chronic stress is much more than a risk factor for lifestyle conditions such as obesity and heart disease. It is the common culprit of low-grade chronic inflammation associated with accelerated aging, decreased immune resilience, and age-related degenerative conditions, such as arthritis, dementia and even cancer."
>
> Ivel De Freitas, MD

the same for my patients. From heart attacks to pneumonias and even autoimmune disease, I noticed that there was almost always this common denominator: stress.

I connected the dots and realized that modern lifestyle was making me and my patients sick; that hypertension, heart disease, diabetes, and even cancer were not the real cause of most of my patients' health challenges, but the consequence of how stress was impacting our body and sabotaging our destiny. I reconnected with why I wanted to become a doctor in the first place and started questioning the status quo. I became again the intellectual rebel I used to be, and I think I have never stopped since.

Discovering the Healing Power of Love

My next wake-up call came while I was doing my internal medicine residency at one of the Yale University programs at Danbury Hospital.

By that time, I thought I had mastered the art of modern medicine. I was just chosen as the chief resident, and I was even a physician advisor for our senior attending to help them optimize their billing and Medicare rule compliance. My specialty was how to get my patients "well enough" to leave the hospital as soon as possible. How to treat patients efficiently and get them happy while still saving money for the system. I had to help decide who met criteria for hospitalization and who could be treated at home. Who needed intensive care and who could be admitted to the regular floor. And, sad but true, how to stay out of trouble by practicing defensive medicine, which has become one of most delicate ethical topics of modern medicine. I was still a good person, and my patients liked me very much, but I was always the doctor in the equation, even on those times when the universe tried to remind me about my human vulnerabilities, here and there, on those occasions when I got sick or I was pregnant. However, I always felt like I was in control, like "I got this" because I was always, even on those days, playing the doctor role. However, that was going soon to change.

Everything started after I took my nine-month-old baby, Anthony, to his regular pediatric checkup. The doctor said he heard irregularities in Anthony's heart rhythm. He confirmed it with an EKG and then recommended an echocardiogram. A few days later we were at the cardiology office and got the worst news I had ever received—my baby had a congenital heart malformation that needed to be fixed immediately. During the following two weeks, we traveled back and forth to New York to complete the extensive preoperative workup needed at Columbia Presbyterian. While my anxiety mounted, I managed to be present and grateful for the resources that we had available that allowed us to bring him to one of the best hospitals on Earth to get his heart fixed. In the meantime, I continued working full-time at the hospital because I would have to take some days off after his surgery.

Surgery day finally arrived. My anxiety and fear reached its highest point when I had to put Anthony on the stretcher on his way to the operating room. Thankfully everything went great, and he was transported to the ICU for monitoring.

The first night was the hardest as Anthony kept moaning from pain every time he breathed in. Despite pain medication being adjusted multiple times, his moaning never subsided until the very next day after he was extubated and finally placed in my arms. This is probably one of the defining moments of my life. There it was. My little one finally was content despite his wounds, chest tube, and IV lines. I hugged him softly and cried, so grateful. And to my joyful surprise, this seemed to help ease his pain. Anthony's moaning stopped, his warm little presence calmed my

LOVE

NOUN - [luhv]

The highest form of nourishing energy, essential for beings to thrive. In the pure frequency of love lies the secret path for oneness. Love is all; all is you.

fears and brought the hope I needed to continue. It was a real healing moment not only for me but for all of us. It was like time had stopped, and we were just one: baby, mom and dad. Anthony's operation changed us deeply and for the better. This was one of the first times that I became aware of the biological and healing power of love. It was also the first time I experienced being a patient, which will change forever the way I empathize with others, especially with my patients.

Things went great; and after two nights in the hospital, we were able to go back home and move on.

However, five months later I got a call from my mom. She was crying while she told me she was diagnosed with breast cancer. She needed surgery. The biopsy wasn't done properly, so I wanted to make sure she was well taken care of for the next steps she needed to take. I invited her to come to Danbury Hospital in Connecticut, where I was working at the time. Shortly after her arrival, she successfully underwent surgery.

She recovered very well. But I was not comfortable with what I was seeing in medicine anymore. I felt we should be doing a better job.

My humanity was awakened by these events, and my empathy started reacting against the system. I began questioning my profession, the scientific method, and everything I had learned in medical school.

I wondered how this could have happened, how these two healthy individuals were sentenced to such a destiny. What could have been the cause of these two incidents, and how could I have helped them stay healthy and beat the statistics?

I also wondered how this could have been prevented, looking for ways to help others to avoid going through what we had gone through.

I learned a lot. I learned there was much more than just hormone replacement and breast cancer, that stress and nutrition as well as environmental toxins could increase the risk of breast cancer and relapse. I learned about the importance of detoxification and methylation pathways to prevent unwanted hormonal and toxic effects. I also learned that toxins, such as pesticides, affect babies' development while in the uterus, and I have supported organic food and the green movement ever since.

Time to Really Wake Up

It is estimated that over eighty thousand chemicals are currently used in the United States. It has been estimated that many of us carry over seven hundred contaminants within our bodies.

Evidence of heavy metals, plastics, phthalates, and pesticides have been reported not only in adults, but even in children as early as at birth, demonstrating that exposure and accumulation start as early as in the uterus.

Where are these toxins coming from?

First of all, it's important to recognize that toxins can come from outside or be created inside your body.

The natural degradation of hormones and different waste products, like lactic acid and CO_2, needs to be eliminated in order to keep your microenvironment—the space where your cells are living and functioning within your own body—clean and your biomolecular core working optimally.

A variety of detox practices have been cultivated and used for centuries by different cultures and civilizations to facilitate and enhance natural elimination processes of the human body. But detox is still considered complementary and even unnecessary by some doctors.

Considered just a health fad, little is taught about it in medical school and formal traditional medical training. Unfortunately, most of what was

> **MICROENVIROMENT**
>
> NOUN [ˈmīkrōənˌvīrənmənt]
>
> The biomolecular nourishing space where your cells are living, functioning and thriving within your own body.
>
> THE ONOGEN DICTIONARY

known back then and even what we know today in this field is empiric, based on old traditions, granny's advice, common sense, and scattered science, so there is no space for it in our curriculum.

It is not that I did not hear about pesticides in my training at all. In fact, I did! But what I learned was that pesticides, heavy metals like lead, and other environmental toxins have been found to be a common factor for rare conditions, such as aplastic anemias, different neurodegenerative disorders, including Parkinsonism, and even some rare leukemias. End of discussion, that was it.

Chelation (a kind of cleansing of the blood of toxins) was superficially mentioned sometimes for severe lead toxicity cases that were presented as rare as well.

As a result, I did not read about the topic again until my son was diagnosed with his heart condition, and I was trying to figure out why he might have gotten it and how I could better help him or other children like him.

I was surprised when I learned that association with pesticides, found in most fruits and vegetables, has been broadly described as a one of the possible causes of congenital problems, such as heart anomalies.

I'm not saying that I was not exposed to this knowledge during medical school. What I am saying is there was no emphasis placed on these kinds of risk factors; no discussions about how to avoid toxin exposures; no discussions on how to help the body's detoxification mechanism work better; no discussion of how we as leaders in the health field should support environmental protection and create more awareness of the subject.

Despite being a highly educated doctor, I was struck by the fact that the healthy food I strived to eat during my pregnancy and my efforts to avoid well-known toxins, such as secondhand smoking, alcohol, and caffeine, were not enough because the vegetables I was eating could have been contaminated with toxins that may have affected my baby. Time to wake up and, again, question the status quo!

Learning to Think Outside the Box

Shortly after all these events, I became severely ill. Everything started with a sore throat—mouth sores—that evolved to severe pain when swallowing, weight loss, and fever for a few weeks. After an extensive workup and weeks of uncertainty, I was diagnosed with a viral infection.

Herpes, the same virus that usually causes cold sores, had taken me while my immune system was severely depressed and had affected my mouth, throat, and esophagus. I could barely swallow for a few weeks, so I lost a lot of weight. My colleagues and I thought I might have cancer because my immunosuppression was so severe. More workup was needed to rule out those possibilities, and I finally recovered.

So now the question was, "Why?" Why did a healthy young woman get so sick in such a short period of time?

In the quest for the answer to these questions, I sought more training, this time outside the box. What I did not know at that time was that I was getting into an area that would revolutionize forever the way I live and practice medicine.

It was during my training at Harvard Medical School in Mind Body Medicine that I heard for the first time the concept of self-care and real prevention. From Dr. Herbert Benson, I learned that our traditional approach to patient care was missing an important piece that would explain the huge American healthcare crisis.

Dr. Benson's theory was based on the concept that to be able to deliver health under the current medical system, medicine should be delivered following a three-legged model. One leg depends on Pharmaceutical Therapies, the second leg depends on Surgery and Medical Procedures, and the third leg depends on Self-Care. He maintained that our system was failing because of the lack of self-care and more efforts needed to be directed to empower and motivate patients to become more active players in their own healing process.

I left convinced that I needed to develop better strategies to motivate my patients and myself to prioritize self-care. Now you understand why I became a biohacking advocate, as you know I am convinced that biohacking is the modern expression of self-care.

However, at that time, my younger self soon realized there were not many tools to support self-care initiatives. By that time, most of the advances in technology and research were applied to the first two legs—pharma and medical devices—and almost none to the third one: self-care.

I came to the profound realization that despite being a physician and a role model of health for my colleagues, family, and friends, my own health and self-care was at the bottom of my own priorities, way below family, profession, and finances. And this was not only me but everyone else I knew within my closest circle.

How could we help our healthcare system to reshape and correct this error if we were the first to miss this important factor in our own lives?

I grew fascinated with this concept and started to research strategies and programs within my hospital to promote and create awareness of the importance of practicing self-care, not only in patients but in healthcare providers as well. I understood for the first time that one of the most important flaws of the healthcare system approach was affecting providers as well.

These new perspectives sparked profound changes in the way I live and practice medicine. They also reconnected me with why I became a doctor in the first place.

I realized that traditional medical training and practice mainly focuses on the "how"—cultivating knowledge and skills through memorization, imitation, and practice. As a result, after a few years, we easily miss the meaning and purpose of our profession, the "why." In my case, these realizations came just in time to rekindle my passion for medicine and understand a hidden healthcare crisis: healthcare providers' burnout.

I understood now why medical school and stress had changed me and how in that process I lost my purpose and my enthusiasm. I understood why I had to sometimes drag myself to work, the same work that I initially had felt so passionate about.

It was at this time that I began to develop research, strategies, and programs within my hospital to promote and create awareness on the importance of practicing self-care—not only in patients but in healthcare providers as well. Part of this program was a progressive online platform to track and support users' positive and healthy lifestyle choices.

CHAPTER 2

Connecting the Dots

Stress has been declared the twenty-first- century epidemic. We live in a chronically stressed culture. Most of us exist in a state of "always ON," near-constant overwork—overwhelmed, tired, and wired. All this stress is taking a serious toll on society.

Many of my patients may look like they have it all, but more often than not their main complaints are a consequence of how chronically sustained their stress is and their tendency to neglect their essential needs. In today's world, we may have different backgrounds, education, status, and wealth, but we all certainly share the same biology that sustains us through the stress of daily living. And that is also key for our gene expression, making us who we are.

You must be thinking now, "Gene expression? Really?"

Yes, really! Stress happens to be very expensive for your biomolecular core, and by affecting that, it also can significantly impact gene expression and your health and longevity.

It also has been reported and is now broadly recognized that up to 90 percent of all visits to primary care doctors are for stress-related complaints. The approach to this is still mainly to label the problem with a diagnosis and treat it with a drug that cools down the symptoms, but that rarely addresses the real source of the problem.

Adding Fuel to the Fire

Between 1996 and 2013, the number of adults prescribed anti-anxiety drugs in the class that includes Xanax (alprazolam) or Ativan (lorazepam)—known as benzodiazepines—rose by 67 percent. Over the same period, the amount of these drugs that was actually dispensed more than tripled, according to a 2016 study.

Today, one in six Americans takes some kind of psychiatric drug—most often antidepressants. Between 1999 and 2008 the number of Americans taking antidepressants also increased by nearly 65 percent. The chronic stress epidemic keeps rising while our therapeutic tools and approaches fail to evolve.

Stress and anxiety are not new to humans. For centuries, people in cultures around the world treasured various herbs, strategies, or both, to help the body to better cope with stress; however, it seems that the therapeutic path our society has chosen is not solving the problem but fueling it.

The opioid epidemic continues to rise, leading to hospitalization and deaths. Society is looking for alternatives, which explains to some extent the increased interest in herbs and ancient practices, such as meditation and yoga, that we have seen in recent years in Western culture. Medicinal herbs such as ashwagandha, ginseng, and rhodiola, and methods based on praying, chanting, breathing, meditation, qigong, tai chi, and yoga are filling a gap well recognized by a sector of our modern Western society. A sector that recognizes the potential dramatic effect of this epidemic and is wise enough to accept ancient wisdom as a potential source of natural alternatives and potential breakthroughs. If we would do this more often, we would all discover how wise our ancestors were and how arrogant and foolish we have become.

It's time to wake up! We all know that stress is here to stay. But, in fact, this is not a bad thing. Stress, well understood, brings more positives than negatives. And well-managed stress can help you to thrive and evolve faster and perform at a higher level.

I'm sure you have experienced what is sometimes called being "wired," that feeling of maximum alertness and focus that characterizes the hormone balance change that is initiated when your stress response system gets activated. That feeling of alertness and sharpness that you probably have experienced when you are working on a project that you feel passionate about. The same feeling many people are looking to recreate or enhance by using amphetamines, hallucinogens, and even small doses of acid (LSD). That feeling that you get when you knock out anxiety and fear, becoming confident of your abilities and in control of your destiny. What some call being at the top of your game.

This happens thanks to a delicate chemical balance mainly regulated between your brain and your adrenals, a small gland located on top of the kidney that produces hormones like cortisol, adrenaline (epinephrine), and norepinephrine that help you to respond adequately to stress. Therefore, the system that modulates your stress response and allows you to perform at the top of your game at any given time is known as the brain-adrenal axis or hypophysis-pituitary-adrenal axis (HPA axis).

An adequate hormone production associated with stress response and a balanced and harmonic biomolecular core are all essential for a healthy stress response—and ultimately for your capacity for coping and your overall performance and success in anything you are trying to accomplish.

But the question is how can you hold this momentum? How can you keep yourself performing at your peak? Wouldn't it be great to be able to hold it and display it the same way every day? But it does not happen that way, does it? What do you have to do to stay at that level, at the top of your game for longer and even in your everyday life?

The answer based on my personal and clinical experience, after my many years of research and nonstop search, lies in your biomolecular core. If you can keep refueling your biomolecular core with exactly what you need—which is not for most people just protein, vegetables, coffee, a few vitamin pills, and meditation—then you may hold this status longer and longer. You can develop this until you have the endurance to hold it and use it every time you need it, just like what you do with your cell phone—just pulling it out of your pocket and using it at its full power any and every time you want.

However, if you do not know how to recharge your system, which is unique for everyone, you are not going to be able to refuel your biomolecular core correctly. And this will compromise not only your performance and health, but your capacity to cope with stress. In other words, if you are walking around with a partially depleted biomolecular core, you are decreasing your chance to succeed and weakening your chance of recovery, which eventually can get you into a dangerous downward spiral. Poorly managed stress can become your worst enemy and a real killer.

As soon as I connected the dots and realized that stress was one of the most common denominators triggering most of the health crises, not only in my life but also in my patients' lives, I embarked on a journey to find ways to stress-proof myself and my patients and to find a formula to allow all of us, myself included, to tolerate stress and take advantage of all the great opportunities this tolerance-enhanced capacity can bring. A personalized formula that helps your body, mind, and spirit stay at the top of your game, bringing you to your real best shape, your *beyond well*.

On Becoming Stress-Proof

Can you really defeat the adverse effects of stress and start to use stress for your own benefits?

Stress has the potential to inspire and motivate you to move toward a goal. This means stress can be good sometimes. Stress well-managed and balanced has the potential to become a kind of personal, virtual motivational coach. However, you must learn how to utilize its pros and mitigate its cons in order to enjoy its benefits and become immune to its drawbacks. This is what I call becoming stress-proof.

This idea was inspired by the lessons I learned from some of my patients facing deadly conditions who shared with me their fears and hopes. For them to share their valuable time and wisdom, while entrusting me to help them through those difficult times, was a privilege. These patients have become mentors and are an eternal inspiration for my lifework.

One of the main lessons I learned from them is that people see what they want to see, and what they see may not be the same that you or anybody else sees. Perception of what is happening is as unique as every individual life, story, feelings, and cultural background.

Therefore, some of my terminally ill patients have taught me how human beings have the capacity to bring the best out of every situation. They have learned how to focus on what they can still enjoy and not on what they have lost or may be losing soon.

I have had patients who are capable of perceiving their disease as an opportunity to thrive, grow, and learn. Despite their suffering they are still capable of showing hope and gratitude. On the other hand, I have met patients going through the same scenario, or even much less serious ones, who are not capable of pulling themselves together, who are defeated even before starting to fight. I have had patients who were going through the worst crisis of their life, and they were still capable of managing highly demanding jobs and family responsibilities. They lived in a highly resilient state, grateful for their job and even cheerful about their life. From these superhumans I heard things like: "I won't quit anything that keeps me going, including my job, because I love it"; "I cannot walk or dance, but I can still talk and laugh"; or "I know I might die soon, but I'm going to give a hell of a fight." On the other hand, I have had patients with less responsibility and less critical situations appear on the verge of a nervous breakdown, triggered by something that for another person would not be stressful at all.

What I have learned is that stress is completely subjective, and its effect on health depends completely on an individual's perception. Perception is based on beliefs, assumptions, values, and conditioning. A situation can be perceived as highly stressful by someone, and not trigger any fear or emotion at all for someone else. Stress does not always arise from an actual threat but from something you perceive as a threat. If you perceive something as stressful, your brain and adrenals release hormones into the blood. If the threat is a tiger that is about to eat you, these hormones may help save your life, making you run faster and fight harder. If the threat is not real, but a virtual concern about any regular daily life issues such as being late for work or not having enough time to finish a project, the same hormones flow through your bloodstream causing an increase in your heart rate, blood pressure, and alertness.

In the book, *Why Zebras Don't Get Ulcers*, Stanford University biologist Robert M. Sapolsky explains how social phenomena, such as social status and poverty, trigger biological stress responses that chronically lead to increased risk of disease and disability. The name of the book is derived from Sapolsky's practical metaphor that I have been using for many years in my practice to explain the difference between episodic and chronic stress. The metaphor starts when a hungry tiger spots a group of zebras on the savannah. The zebras notice the tiger, turning *on* their stress response system. As the fight-or-flight hormone response switches on, the brain-adrenal axis orchestrates changes in their physiology that help them increase their chances of survival. The zebras begin to run for their lives. Finally, the tiger catches one zebra, and the rest of the zebras relax, and they go back to their peace of mind, relaxation mode. I explain to my patients that this is the best example of how stress is meant to help us survive.

However, humans' brains are wired differently, as we have the capacity to connect emotionally with the event and are also preoccupied with and planning for the future. Our stress response usually stays *on* instead of fading away. I explain this using a different metaphor, by imagining if the zebras thought like us. They would empathize with the zebra that just died, with his/her family, and they would also think about the chances another tiger would come or that the tiger would get hungry again in a few days and would come back for another zebra.

The metaphor becomes stronger when we understand that the tigers in our daily life are due dates, traffic jams, micronutrient deficiencies, alcohol, drugs and medications, chronic inflammation, chronic pain, environmental toxins, and even financial, professional, and relationship expectations. Every time you or your body face these challenges your biomolecular core may get hit as if you are facing a tiger that is about to eat you, depending upon your perception of the challenge and your biomolecular core reserve.

So now I ask: What are the tigers in your life? I want you to understand that your own tigers can be perceived by somebody else as a kitty cat. It depends on how confident you feel about being prepared and in control of the outcome that are your tigers. Remember, you cannot control the tiger, but you can control your perception and how well prepared you feel to face it. Understanding this allows you to create a strategy that is key to giving you back a sense of control and helping to better manage or even dissipate your fears.

When you feel you have control of what is happening you feel empowered—you can dominate the tigers in your life, and eventually those tigers become kitty cats. When this happens, new tigers will be born as your path elevates. This means you need to move on and master and dominate those new tigers. You need to keep growing and use your own stress for your own benefit, until you finally master the stress-proof status that we should all enjoy. This is a practice that is usually mastered by famous entrepreneurs and leaders who have achieved massive success in their fields. It is not that the accomplishment nourished them at the end of the journey. In fact, the challenges and tigers they have faced on the path have kept them motivated to move and conquer new horizons.

Do you have any idea of how high your perception of your personal stress level is at this point in time? Please answer these two questions using the provided scale and reflect on your responses and how you can start working on your perception to help you improve your stress management.

1. How often do you feel that you are unable to control the important things in your life?
   Never _____ Almost Never _____ Sometimes _____
   Fairly Often _____ Very Often _____

2. How often do you feel you are on top of things and that you can control your destiny?
   Never _____ Almost Never _____ Sometimes _____
   Fairly Often _____ Very Often _____

These are questions I have taken from The Perceived Stress Scale (PSS), a tool developed to help us understand individual stress perception. If you are curious, you can fill it out at https://onogen.com/immunity-age-quiz/ and get an objective and validated measurement of your stress level.

From Bad to Worse: "Always On" Mode to "Power Saver" Mode

Our stress response is not meant to stay on for too long without breaks to slow down and recharge. Chronic stress increases your energy use, which increases your micronutrients use, which can potentially create a supply-demand mismatch opening significant gaps on your biomolecular core. Higher use means higher needs. If you ignore signs your biomolecular core is getting depleted—decreased energy, mood, and brain clarity—you are ignoring that your reserves are wearing off; you are ignoring that you have significant gaps in your biomolecular core and biological foundation, and that your body is going to perform poorly. This decrease in performance, which is usually not taken seriously by physicians, is a subtle signal that your body is trying to warn you there is a problem.

When your biomolecular core reserve wears off, your day-to-day performance—energy, mood, joy, brain clarity, and sex drive, i.e., your quality of life—gets compromised, along with your health and longevity.

The wearing down of your biomolecular core sets your cells to a status of "power-saver mode." As with your computer or mobile phones, when the battery is running down some functions shut or slow down to save power for the main functions of the device. When your body goes into power-saver mode, something very similar happens. Your biomolecular core shuts or slows down some processes to save resources for the most essential, life-sustaining ones.

Like when a device goes on power-saver mode and the screen is not as bright and the processing speed slows, something similar happens to you. Your mood and outlook on life are not as bright, your brain clarity and task-processing speed slows down, as does your capacity to multitask. I'm pretty sure you have probably felt like that sometime in your life. We all have.

This is explained by accumulative micronutrient deficiencies that progressively weaken your biomolecular core, preventing you from running on full-power mode. This is reflected in your capacity to enjoy optimal energy, mood, brain clarity, sleep, sex drive, health, longevity, and performance.

Being in power-saver mode prevents you from achieving your highest mental and physical performance potential, making it more challenging to cope with stress. Running on power-saver mode weakens your natural coping and recovery mechanism and worsens your perception of the situation. This perpetuates a vicious cycle that can turn you into your own worst enemy and sabotage your efforts to achieve your goals.

As I see it, negativity, repetitive thoughts, depression, anxiety, chronic fatigue, low energy, foggy brain, insomnia, and decreased sex drive are most of the time signals that your biomolecular core imbalances are exceeding acceptable levels. These are all signs you are developing important gaps within your biomolecular core.

The main challenge in medicine today is that if we evaluate you using standard laboratory tests, most of the time we can't find any abnormalities that would alert us to a problem and would allow us to be proactive. These gaps do not manifest on the traditional labs until the level of imbalances in the core build up enough to start compromising more essential pathways or processes; this can be manifested as high blood pressure, high blood sugar, frequent colds, high cholesterol or triglycerides, elevated liver enzymes, elevated inflammatory markers, hormone imbalances, thyroid problems, and many others. If these alert signals are treated with medications following the standards of care principles in current medicine, patients may experience relief or improvement to some degree. However, the source of the problem—a rundown biomolecular core—continues building up, perpetuating the problem and eventually affecting vital processes such as immune function, cellular and tissue regeneration, and DNA repair and maintenance. This chain of events can eventually activate uncontrolled inflammation and degenerative processes, triggering—depending on your genetic predisposition—autoimmunity, heart disease, dementia, cancer, and other age-related degenerative conditions.

I learned through my research and clinical experience that by improving your biomolecular balance you can dramatically decrease your stress level. By rebalancing your biomolecular core, mood and thinking processes also get rebalanced. I have hypothesized that by replenishing the biomolecular core with exactly what it is missing, we can help people cope with stress in a more efficient way and get them to play at the top of their game.

As we have discussed, stress depends on perception. But by fueling your biomolecular core correctly, you increase your chances of facing adversity in a more positive mode. Like when you are preparing for a camping trip and you take everything you may possibly need to survive, when you are facing stress and you get there with all the resources, you'll be automatically more relaxed than if you lack resources.

You need to decide if you are going to face your next challenge with your body status in scarcity and survival mode or in a recharged and optimal mode, either on power-saver mode or full-power mode, or what we call today in my practice your PRIME mode. This, my friends, influences your perception of stress *big time*. With a fully charged, primed, biomolecular core, your brain and neurotransmitters run at their highest potential, allowing you to face situations in a more objective way and avoid the distorted thinking that most humans have a tendency to experience in such situations, especially when they are tired or not in their best shape.

How would you rather face your next challenge? On power-saver mode or on full-power, PRIME mode?

Just as when you have to perform a task and are sleep-deprived or super-tired, a task that might be easy for you otherwise might seem harder than it really is. So, imagine that although you might not feel hungry or starving or depleted, your brain and biomolecular core are. When your thinking is distorted, you may exaggerate perceived shortcomings, causing you to paint events far worse than they actually are. Recharging your biomolecular core and providing your brain with all the necessary biomolecular factors can help you to cope with stress better and prevent distorted thinking.

Burnout: When the Doctor Is Sick Too

While on my own path to optimize my health, I became a wellness advocate. I ate healthy, I quit dairy and gluten, and even animal protein for a while. I ran and exercised at least four to five times a week. I have finished different races and half-marathons, and I have an established personal yoga and meditation practice. Nevertheless, despite my lab results and physicals being consistent with the best health status someone like me could have, I did not feel great; in fact, I felt exhausted. I thought I was depressed, but I was not willing to take drugs for it. I kept having occasional health crises usually related to or just after periods of high stress. It was then, while I was working as a hospitalist, on a seven-on-seven-off, twelve-hour shift schedule, while teaching residents and growing my private practice on the side at the same time, with very little help, and playing the role of perfect loving wife and mom, when I had another one of my wake-up call. I got burned out, *extremely and for real!*—despite knowing all I knew, meditating almost on a daily basis, eating healthy, and exercising consistently.

Stress affects all of us. It has not spared healthcare providers. In fact, it is eroding and slowly debilitating our healthcare system from within. A recent study found that up to 69 percent of healthcare providers reported having experienced at least one symptom of burnout.

People affected by burnout from work-related stress may experience physical, mental, and emotional exhaustion, and present with some or all of the following symptoms:

- Fatigue and low energy
- Foggy brain
- Low sex drive
- Low or blue mood
- Depression
- Negative and repetitive thinking
- Decreased coping capacity
- Reduced performance and productivity
- Anxiety
- Emotional detachment
- Feeling listless
- Difficulty concentrating
- Lack of creativity
- Negative attitudes towards self and others
- Low commitment to the role
- Loss of purpose
- Irritability or quickness to anger
- Cynicism
- Emotional numbness
- Frustration and resentment

Work-related stress, becoming burned out and feeling overwhelmed to the point of ill health due to the demands of your job or work environment can happen to any employee, in any job, and at any age or stage of professional life.

In my case and that of my colleagues, the rise in healthcare costs, progressive cuts to reimbursements, and a challenging healthcare business model, where providers are rewarded more by volume of patients, rather than the quality of the service provided, has precipitated what is being called an epidemic. An epidemic that is debilitating not only to healthcare as an institution, but leaving physicians exhausted, skeptical, and frustrated, and patients feeling disappointed, abandoned, cheated, and resentful.

In the meantime, stress and burnout are still not considered a clinical diagnosis. Although this epidemic is taking a toll on all of us—patients and doctors alike—a solution has not been found. We keep ignoring the elephant in the room. Stress is an unavoidable factor that can impact our lives positively or negatively, but if we ignore it and refuse to learn to manage it, we eventually become sick.

This selective blindness prevents most of us from seeing and recognizing the magnitude and the scope of this insidious epidemic. All the factors of current medical practice mentioned above leave very little room for most providers to look for solutions.

We often hear complaints about physicians lacking compassion and empathy. Looking at the whole picture, it's easy to understand how the healthcare system and academia push compassion and empathy to the side.

In a culture that promotes self-neglecting behaviors such as skipping meals, sleep deprivation, and a "do-not-cry-ever" policy, how do we now want physicians to display empathy and compassion? How can we ask physicians to empathize with others when they can barely empathize with themselves?

The system is broken, and this is not just me saying this. Great minds in the fields of altruism like Dr. Stephen G. Post recognize it as well. Dr. Post is a renowned researcher, public speaker, and best-selling author dedicated to the science of altruism and compassion. He is the founding director of the Center for Medical Humanities, Compassionate Care, and Bioethics at Stony Brook University in the School of Medicine, Department of Preventive Medicine. His main research is focused on the ways in which giving, empathy, and compassion can enhance not only the health, well-being, and professional satisfaction of the healthcare professional, but patient outcomes. His science and wealth of knowledge make him, in my opinion, one of the most knowledgeable minds in the field.

I, in fact, had the privilege of meeting with him a few times while we were planning the first symposium on the science of love. In one of those meetings, he shared with me that he was leading a project to incorporate classes in empathy and compassion into the medical curriculum. I know he has been successful in his quest, and thanks to his unconditional effort he has spread this concept to multiple medical schools.

This is just one sign that awareness is slowly rising; however, we all know we need much more than that to create meaningful change. We need to continue working together.

How can we ask healthcare professionals to be compassionate to others if they get zero or minimal compassion from their working environment or from their colleagues and patients? To make things harder, healthcare providers face their patients in a trying environment—not always well-rested, fed, and relaxed, but most commonly exhausted, frustrated and sometimes even resentful. They face their patient not at the top of their game. This is a problem! No wonder errors happen more often than they should.

To foster a more empathetic and compassionate culture within our healthcare system, we need to break the "if you feel tired, just keep going," "if you are hungry, wait, " "if you want to pee, hold it," "if you want to cry, don't you dare" paradigms. Otherwise, things won't ever change. If you haven't eaten or taken a break all day, and it seems that nobody cares about you, what are the odds that you could empathize with the patient whose food came thirty minutes late and complains to you about it?

Healthcare providers are overworked and under-rested most of the time. They are also under constant pressure, constantly reminded of the risk of malpractice liability—even when trying to prevent patients from undergoing unnecessary tests, and being required to follow strict guidelines and standard of care dictated by academia and medical boards over their clinical judgement. This unfortunately promotes increasing malpractice concerns, which further impact the capacity for these individuals to practice empathy and compassion. These challenges are associated with the deleterious concept of defensive medicine that has transformed the doctor-patient relationship deeply, from a bilateral trustworthy relationship to a faithless one.

It should not be surprising that we are facing a healthcare crisis as we now know that most of our providers are already unhappy or unsatisfied with the practice of medicine.

We are not going to fix this just by teaching doctors how to breathe and meditate. In order to start experiencing a real change, a profound culture change needs to happen. Patients and doctors alike need to feel that the system is designed to care for them, that the system prioritizes their well-being. They need to learn that human well-being and self-care should never be sacrificed in pursuit of academic, financial, or hierarchy achievement.

This is not to be taught in a classroom. This should be taught in the hospital halls, at the bedside of each patient, and in each and every one of their classes that addresses human nature. My hope is that the crisis we are going through right now is an opportunity to awaken and empower all of us, to start taking advantage of every opportunity to remind ourselves that we all are trying to do our best. And by practicing compassion and unconditional love with ourselves and others we can start seeing those changes happen within healthcare and academia soon. We can collaborate and become a catalyst for this needed change that not only needs to take place within medical schools but within society as well.

I invite you to join the movement of making kindness, empathy, and compassion go viral. Don't you think there is more of a chance to do that now? Remember, change always starts within ourselves.

Most of the physicians and healthcare providers I know are trying to put their best face forward and display empathy, compassion, and kindness towards their patients. This is especially noticeable when they are well-rested at the beginning of their shift. Physicians are usually nice by nature, but emotional exhaustion can make even the nicest person cranky. So don't take that smile and kind gesture from your doctor for granted.

Despite focusing on physician burnout, this epidemic is affecting everyone. I have seen it in young, successful, and talented adults, entrepreneurs, lawyers, celebrities, firefighters, law enforcement, teachers, employees of all different fields and stay-at-home parents. Burnout does not respect age, gender, race, or profession and appears in all groups with the same three main components:

- Emotional exhaustion: "I am exhausted."
- Depersonalization: "I have become bitter, cynical, and very skeptical."
- Reduced personal accomplishment: "I've lost my purpose."

If you feel tired all the time, drained from whatever you do, if you sometimes feel too tired to care, you have a hard time empathizing with people or getting up in the morning to do what you need to do, or you don't feel excited about what you do anymore, you are probably exhibiting some signs of burnout and need to start doing something about it. You should start by going to your doctor and getting a traditional checkup first.

My Own Path Out of Burnout

As I said before, I am talking from my own experience here, as I became burned out myself. At the time I was working a twelve-hour shift in a very busy community hospital in South Florida with a very demanding population. I was also growing my lifestyle medicine practice, participating in a Functional Medicine Fellowship and raising a family. Burnout did not spare me despite my good efforts and my well-intentioned behavior and lifestyle. I ate right and exercised and meditated on a regular basis. I enjoyed my work at the hospital, and I loved everything I was doing, but getting out of bed in the morning started to become harder. Despite sleeping well, it seemed to me that I was having a hard time recovering. I noticed this pattern especially after day three of my seven-day shifts. I still managed to pull myself together with exercise, coffee, and positive affirmations and get through my day looking put-together. My colleagues and students admired me for my capacity to smile and move along from any challenging patient encounter. There were many—most people lying in a hospital bed are not especially thrilled about being there. They're typically going through tremendous amounts of stress themselves.

I was one of those doctors called to manage the most complex, demanding patients because I was described then as having unlimited patience and amazing empathy. Little did they know. I used to take breathing breaks during my rounds, usually short ones in between each patient and a longer one in the middle of my day. I also tried to recharge myself with positive energy during those breaks to be able to deliver myself at the top of my game to every one of my patients. I have always believed that positive energy, love, and hope are very important healing tools that we need to present at every encounter. This all sounds great, but keeping this attitude in the trying environment I was in was taking a toll. By the end of my day, I felt completely exhausted and empty, as if all my energy had been sucked out of me. Sometimes I even felt that what I was doing was not worth it.

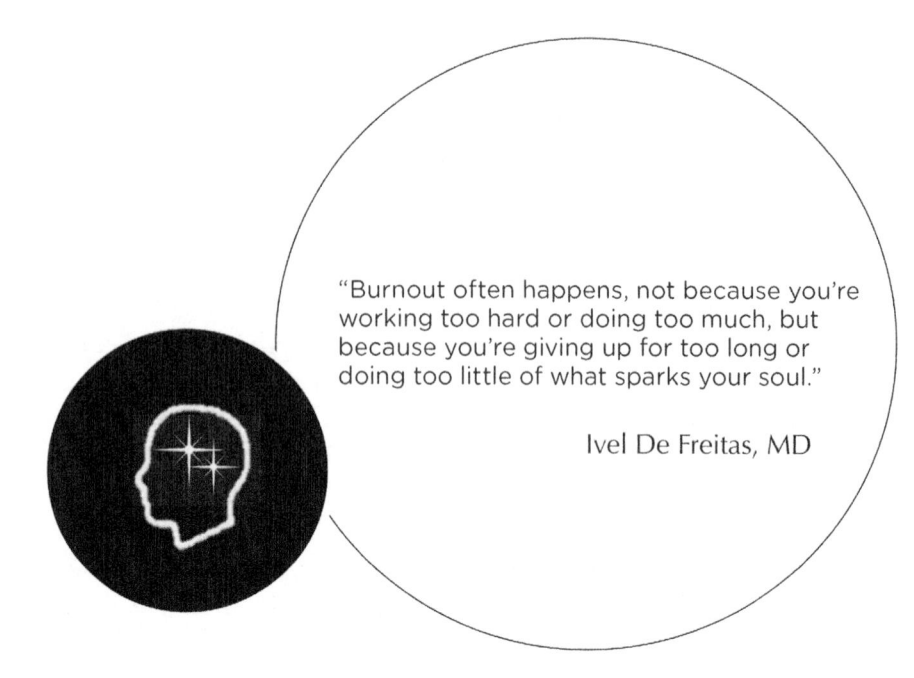

> "Burnout often happens, not because you're working too hard or doing too much, but because you're giving up for too long or doing too little of what sparks your soul."
>
> Ivel De Freitas, MD

What I am describing is what I described before as signs of burnout.

As soon as I realized I was getting burned out, I immersed myself in research and went through thousands of papers looking for options to get myself back in shape. I knew stress was the root of the problem. So, I began working on a plan that would help me to manage stress better and prevent burnout. This project helped rekindle my passion for medicine. Through this project I found a new purpose that lighted my soul and helped me to heal.

I ended up learning an important lesson on this journey of overcoming burnout and becoming more stress-proof. Redefining my purpose at that time helped me to rekindle my passion for medicine. Just as couple therapies recommend bringing newness and excitement to get the spark back in a relationship, I found that by applying this strategy to the relationship I had with my job, I resurrected my excitement and enthusiasm, overcoming burnout. Try it, add something exciting to your routine, and see how your spark lights up and your enthusiasm exponentially increases. Since then, I have seen this happen multiple times. By the way, a dear friend and client, Grant Cardone, describes this really well in many of his interviews and social media channels.

Grant insists that people feel burnout when they have either lost focus on their purpose or they are following somebody else's instead of finding and following their own. I think Grant is right on this. I know for a fact that a key part of my patients' total recovery depends on channeling their passions and finding a purpose. However, I would add to this thoughtful observation, based on my years of practice, that the first culprit of most patients is chronic stress first creating a biomolecular supply-demand mismatch that compromises important processes in our biomolecular core. This might result in people feeling fatigue, which contributes to them losing their focus. They forget what they were working for: the why. They lose the drive and the desire to take care of themselves. They become what I call "too tired to care," and unfortunately the first to go then is caring for themselves. They lose their purpose—if they ever had it; they lose their "why." They focus instead on the "what," which creates a vicious cycle that most of the time becomes impossible to break.

Symptoms of burnout are debilitating not only for your body, but also for your mind and spirit. How do you get excited if you can barely feel? It is like being numb. It is like being in darkness, like in a black hole. A black hole that can only be left if you or someone who loves you convinces you there is hope and that it is worth it to look for a way out. In my opinion, what is missing in your biomolecular core is eclipsing your way out of burnout. It is slowing down pathways as important as the ones that produce key neurotransmitters like dopamine and serotonin that are essential for human beings to hope, to believe and get up and move in the right direction.

Learning what your unique needs are and finding ways to meet them consistently are, in my experience, the best first step and, in fact, the foundation for anybody's recovery from burnout. In fact, this first step of upgrading your biology has in my experience a ripple effect that has helped my patients to clarify their mind and redefine their why, which solidifies their healing and recovery from burnout.

Incorporating Love into the Formula

I was in the process of putting my physician burnout pilot study together when I met Stefan Deutsch, a philosopher and psychotherapist from New York. I met him while taking care of his mother in the hospital.

If I concentrate and take a nice deep breath, I can still relive the serenity I felt every time I walked into this patient's room. It was literally something I have never experienced and haven't again to this day. The only thing I can say is that it reminded me of the serenity and peace I feel when I walk into a familiar place, a place where I feel loved. I remember the meditation music, the warm lighting, and the peace and love you could breathe in the air. By walking in, you could literally feel you were transported outside of the hospital to a very special place. I knew they were very special people the first day I walked in that room; it was only later that I learned that life was introducing me to my next mentor.

A week after my daytime shift, I came back for my night-shift week. I met Stefan at the main hospital entrance. He updated me on his mom's status because as of that week I was no longer taking care of her. He also shared with me his professional background and gave me a quick introduction to his pioneering work in human development and nurturing love. He told me that he thought that his work could help providers be more empathetic and happier—he had noticed that the environment was not really conducive to that.

He also told me that he had chosen me because he noticed my energy when I walked in the room. Energy that he thought was also transferred to the residents who were rounding with me. He said he felt this energy was different from the rest of the providers he encountered during his mom's hospital stay. He literally said he felt I was the embodiment of love. That I personified his theory of nurturing love, and the way I behaved with my patients and residents was the best example of what his theory could do for the healthcare crisis.

I was not expecting that! But I added it to my list of "the best compliments ever." As you can imagine, he got my attention. I was already putting together my pilot study with the idea to fight burnout. He was another interesting resource to bring new ideas to the table.

Stefan sent me an email with some thoughts to jump-start our meeting. I am going to share the original email as it woke me up to the importance of self-love, sharing in very simple words his functional and scientifically validated theory of love. I hope that by reading the same words I read that day, I can trigger your curiosity to learn more, follow his work and read his amazing book, *Love Decoded*.

Here is what he wrote:

Meeting with Dr. Ivel De Freitas—Sat. 11-15-14

How does our understanding that love is nourishment help people achieve well-being?

Why don't people who know that certain behaviors of theirs, like overeating, not exercising, smoking, and so on are unhealthy—stop doing them?

Or people who have started new, healthy behaviors—stop them?

Most of us are brought up getting love—which we now know to be life-sustaining nourishment—conditionally, meaning only when we behave in ways that others feel we deserve.

We internalize this message to the point that our inner voice mimics the parents and culture. We come to believe that we don't deserve love from others or from ourselves—unless we are perfect. The final problem people face is that having love come from their environment means they conclude, and their brain neuropathways come to operate with the assumption, that love—loving nourishment—only comes from the environment, just like air, food, and water. Human beings aren't proactively or properly taught to nourish themselves with love. That would be unconditionally—exactly like with air, food, and water.

We will never be good enough to love ourselves, be perfect enough, unless the old paradigm of love as a "soup" of romantic and nurturing feelings and emotions is replaced with the new knowledge that loving energy is nourishment.

The conclusion that brings us to—we don't have to earn it or deserve it—any more than air, food, or water.

To retrain our neuropathways takes time and willpower. Individuals need to be trained:

1. To become aware of their propensity for behaving conditionally with themselves (and others).
2. To work with a vision that it is possible to love oneself and others unconditionally, and it is acceptable to ask for unconditional love in return.
3. To learn to communicate with awareness, vision, and in a loving context.

We work with lists for visioning, awareness of self-talk, framing, and listening skills for communicating more effectively.

We encourage individuals to create one unconditional relationship—not conceptually, but in actuality—using the new definition of love, and the new tools and skills.

> The process can bring to awareness painful, past conditional, unloving behaviors from family and others—as well as one's own unloving behaviors toward self and others.
>
> Once people realize/recognize how much better they feel loving themselves unconditionally, these behaviors begin to be transformed to: Behaving more lovingly with family members, colleagues, friends, patients.
>
> The final piece of the loving puzzle is learning how to not accept unloving behaviors from others, in a firm but loving manner.
>
> RESOURCES—Dr. Ivel De Freitas's approach to wellness; Deutsch's Continuum Theory; Watson's concepts of "Transpersonal Caring"; Fredrickson's research; Dr. Bruce Lipton's concepts on energy; Dr. Gary Schwartz's concepts of energy transference.

This meeting was followed by two years of work and weekly meetings that got me to a higher level of self-awareness and enlightened my path. I could not leave this episode and this special mentor out of this book.

I became my own subject of experimentation, and I tried his theory in my own personal life. I noticed a big difference. As I have done with everything I have encountered in my life that has been enlightening and helped me to thrive, I incorporated it into my practice without any hesitation. My initial goal was exactly what he had mentioned in the letter: it was to motivate my patients to do what they knew they needed to do to get healthier. After all, this is the area where most of the lifestyle and wellness plans and programs are failing. People get started but then quit. "I could not find the time." "I do not have the energy to do it." "I got excited at the beginning, but then life and work got complicated, and I quit."

All this probably sounds familiar to you, doesn't it?

I also merged his theory into my research protocol to promote well-being within the medical community, so he became a co-investigator in my research on physician burnout.

From this experience I learned a lot, and I improved how I managed stress in my life. I became a better wife, mom, doctor, friend, and, in general, a better person. I again highly recommend Stefan's book, *Love Decoded*, to start working on the most important relationship we need to cultivate during our lifespan: the relationship with our inner self.

By embracing his theory of love as essential nourishment—as food, air, and water are—I also became more aware of the biological power of love and oxytocin. Oxytocin is a hormone secreted by the posterior lobe of the pituitary gland, a pea-sized structure at the base of the brain. It's sometimes known as the "cuddle or love hormone," because it is released when people snuggle up or bond. It is also known as the "anti-stress hormone" because it has been associated with meditation and positive emotions such as empathy, kindness, trust, compassion, and love. It is also the main hormone responsible for uterus contractions during childbirth, breast milk "letting down" during breastfeeding, and even orgasm. Oxytocin has also been found to be capable of stimulating stem cells to accelerate tissue regeneration. Several in vitro studies have also proposed that oxytocin could act as a selective natural chemotherapy agent because it has been observed to kill cancer cells.

While different from most chemo drugs, oxytocin stimulates immune system function and tissue regeneration. Oxytocin has also been found to be essential for normal child development and growth, and if there is either, or both, lack of love or oxytocin, child development is compromised. Child abuse and neglect, as well as lack of love, have been well described, and it is today broadly recognized as one of the causes of stunted growth and brain development, just as what happened in childhood malnutrition. There is also evidence suggesting that elevated levels of oxytocin can positively impact gene expression, DNA repair, and cell function.

Therefore, I would like to propose that based on Stefan's theory, validated by Barbara Fredrickson and her renowned scientific work on love—described in her book *Love 2.0: Finding Happiness and Health in Moments of Connection*. Love, meaning nourishing and not romantic love, should be treated as another essential nutrient for our biomolecular core. Although the mechanism is not clear yet, and we are not even close to understanding these processes—which by the way is greatly explained by first, a lack of consensus on the definition of love, and second, by the lack of interest within the scientific community to study this extraordinary subject—we need to keep bringing the subject to the table.

What is clear to me is that love—oxytocin and the biomolecular pathways triggered by it—are as essential to our biomolecular core stability as vitamins, minerals, antioxidants, hormones, and peptides. Therefore, more effort should be made to foster more research and provide education by creating room and encouraging discussions on the science of love. I am also proud to say that the First Symposium of the Science of Love was held in NYC in 2015, organized by Stefan Deutsch, and I had the honor to participate with multiple experts in the field, including Jean Watson, Eva Selhub, Harville Hendrix, and Helen LaKelly Hunt. The foundations are being built for love to become a new scientific truth, and for this new truth to triumph, we need the support of people like you to spread the word.

CHAPTER 3

The Final Breakthrough

The PRIME Concept Was Born

Just as I was working on improving my relationship with my inner self and integrating what I had learned about the benefits of this important nourishing element, love, I met G. This was another of those serendipitous events that seemed to become a repetitive pattern in my life. I was still working as a hospitalist, and my pilot study had been recently approved. G is still my patient, and she has also become my dear friend. She is an amazing woman who supports natural medicine and was for twenty years the manager of a practice in South Florida where the main focus was orthomolecular medicine.

Orthomolecular medicine is a form of alternative medicine aimed at maintaining human health through high intravenous doses of vitamins and nutrients. The concept is built on the idea of an optimum nutritional environment in the body and suggests that diseases reflect deficiencies in this environment. Treatment for disease, according to this philosophy, involves attempts to correct "imbalances or deficiencies based on individual biochemistry" by use of substances such as vitamins, minerals, amino acids, trace elements, and fatty acids. This concept, although practiced by many alternative physicians since the 1970s, and similar to what I have proposed so far in my book, has been the subject of controversy and skepticism. This is mostly explained by the scarcity of sound scientific evidence and the lack of interest from big pharma to study and validate this tool—mainly because the formulas are unpatentable with minimal profit potential for them. Despite the lack of interest from big pharma and negative propaganda, this approach has survived and proven its potential throughout the years, helping millions of patients around the world within the complementary medicine arena.

The Myers' cocktail and high doses of vitamin C and glutathione have been the main tools that these physicians have been using to help their patients, and they are the most broadly tested strategies. So, when I met G, she had just left the practice, and she was looking for a doctor to take care of her and her mom's IV infusions.

Her mom was in her mid-eighties at that time and had been diagnosed with vascular dementia a few years prior. G shared with me that as soon as she was told about her mom's diagnosis she got her mom started on glutathione. She felt the therapy had worked to stop the progression of her mom's cognitive decline. Her mother's doctor had told her he did not understand how she had lasted so long with so little evidence of disease progression or the typical functional deterioration that seems to be common in these types of cases.

Glutathione, the peptide that G's mom was getting, is an important antioxidant that our body makes. Its production progressively declines with aging, and the decline in most people starts as early as in their late-thirties. Different studies linked this natural decline in glutathione production with the increase of oxidative damage that has been associated with aging, aging-related-diseases and natural functional decline. Glutathione is also used as a beauty aid, either given intravenously or orally. Studies suggest that people supplementing with either glutathione or its precursor N-acetylcysteine experienced a skin lightening effect, an increase in turgor and elasticity and decrease of wrinkles; all this is explained by its potent antioxidative and blocking effect on the production of melanin, the natural skin pigment.

Therefore, G was using the same IV therapies that she had signed her mom up for, incorporating it as part of her well-thought-out longevity and anti-aging strategy. I have to confess that G's youthful look and amazing energy together with her mom's health story inspired me to pursue training in the field of IV nutrients, moving from there by my curiosity and adventurous spirit to the field of biomolecular medicine.

Soon after being trained, I started applying the therapies to myself. I mainly focused on the Myers' cocktail and glutathione to start with, just trying to recreate a fundamental, natural, and traditional therapy developed by Dr. John Myers at Johns Hopkins in the 1970s. I began using the same formula as everyone else since the standard "one-size-fits-all" approach has been standard for the practice of medicine since the 1960s and the antibiotic revolution. Despite that, the results for me were impressive enough to catch my attention. As soon as I started getting the therapies, I felt amazingly great. In fact, it made me feel better than I ever imagined I could feel. My skin, my hair, my energy, my brain clarity, my mood, and sex drive were all enhanced. This was a breakthrough for me—I thought that after being a wellness advocate for many years I had already optimized most areas of my life. I was already feeling the best I could ever feel for my chronological age. I was eating right, exercising consistently, and meditating daily. I was also taking supplements and optimizing my detoxification pathways naturally. I had also implemented Deutsch's theory and integrated Buddhist practices on kindness and compassion into my life. I felt like I was at the top of my well-being.

However, it wasn't until I started getting my intravenous biomolecular therapies that I realized there was still room for improvement. That is when I decided to call it PRIME. It seems to me that incorporating this therapeutic modality into my personal wellness plan not only brought me to a state of greatest strength, vigor, and success in my life, but filled the gaps I was missing to really achieve my highest potential, kind of gaining superpowers and becoming supernatural.

Yes, I am serious, although I know it sounds crazy. To my surprise, after getting PRIME I achieved a level of fulfillment that has been key for me moving to a higher vibrational level, where I feel joyous and grateful, the mindset that I enjoy now. A state of mind that allows me to face challenges as if anything is possible, overcoming fear and frustration every day.

I am convinced that for extraordinary results you need extraordinary measures. PRIME for me is that extraordinary approach that has allowed me to continue evolving, getting progressively closer to what I think and propose is the truest and highest expression of myself—not just physically and mentally, but also spiritually. After all, we are all interconnected, so it should not surprise us that our spirituality and soul are also connected to our physical body and benefit from a balanced and strong biomolecular core. Mind, body, and soul, all interconnected and synergistically working together to keep us thriving and growing.

Of course, as my close circle of family and friends witnessed this transformation, they grew curious. I was so enthusiastic that I could not wait to share this revelation with others. So, my husband signed up as my next patient, followed by my parents and then close friends and relatives who were willing to try it. Interestingly enough, all of them experienced the same positive effect when I applied my novel approach to them.

What was shocking to me was that despite reports from thousands of patients and practitioners who have been utilizing this method safely over the last fifty years, and the positive reports published in peer-reviewed medical journals—one of them from Dr. David Katz from Yale University—these therapies were still limited to alternative and complementary medicine practitioners. It is clear to me that the data on it is weak compared to the humongous studies conducted and financed by big pharma, but does it not make sense that priming the body and optimizing its nutritional reserves would be the best way to start approaching any therapeutic plan? Don't we know at this point in time that most Americans do not eat a diet that meets the increased micronutrient demand that modern life imposes on them?

It is true that studies are limited, in early phase, and no resources have been assigned to continue pursuing the development of protocols and more accurate and functional diagnostic tools. But shouldn't common sense prevail, allowing this fascinating field to finally step up to the level it should be? The simple fact that IV vitamins and nutrients are unpatentable has been a significant reason it has not been studied more. No big pharma or big budgets are assigned to these unpatentable tools, no matter how beneficial they can be, in a world where profit is the main incentive to develop therapies and technology. However, the results I have seen in my patients and experienced myself has become my main source of inspiration and courage to keep walking this unpaved path. Inspiration and courage that help me to get to the last two steps for my final breakthrough.

When "One Size" No Longer Fits All

During this whole process is when the whole baseline theory of orthomolecular medicine finally clicked for me. Seeing my clinical results and going back to basic science, it became clear to me that we all have a biomolecular core—a core where trillions of biochemical reactions responsible for the optimal function and expression of our biological and genetic makeup are constantly happening without our awareness. Every little task you do depends on a harmonious balance of these biochemical reactions. Biochemical processes that are essential for your cells to stay healthy and for you to enjoy vibrant energy, happy mood, glowing skin, shiny hair, healthy nails, balanced hormones, strong immune system, great sex, and good working genes. The list of those biomolecular factors you need to keep the wheel rolling are: micronutrients, amino acids, minerals, and specific antioxidants and peptides that are essential for your body's optimal performance. Just as a lack of material in a factory creates gaps and a defective final product, deficiencies of some of these factors create gaps in your biomolecular core, compromising your overall performance and health.

Broadly adopting the innovative concept of a biomolecular core as the functional micronutrient reserve of the cells will accelerate this fascinating field and rebuild healthcare's foundation to embrace the innovative concepts of genomics, artificial intelligence, and personalized biomolecular medicine. This is a concept that will allow medicine to move from a disease management model to a real healthcare model. Where medicine not only helps you to stay healthy but also supports you in your own personal journey to become the best expression of yourself in each and every single area of personal development.

I discovered that filling those specific gaps that are keeping you away from your *beyond well* state is not easy. What I found shook my entire belief system—at least the one I created after going through medical school. I learned that despite following a great nutritious diet and supplementation regimen, most of us are still not getting close to meeting all of our biomolecular needs. Subtle deficiencies of these important factors significantly impact your cellular function. As the cells adjust to these subtle deficiencies they shut down noncritical pathways to keep the critical ones from failing. As in a factory, when you have to close some production lines, the final product may come up defective or it may take longer to make, making the process less efficient.

The same happens with your body. As your cells shut down some pathways, some of your functions might get compromised, not necessarily to a level that can cause disease, but to a level that can decrease your natural abilities to perform, feel happy, heal, and keep your immune system protecting you against infections. These subtle biomolecular gaps may translate into symptoms such as low energy, foggy brain, moods swings, decreased sex drive, and frequent colds. Symptoms that most doctors just do not really get concerned about, as our mindset is trained more towards finding a complex diagnosis with a technical name.

While going through this breakthrough, I also learned that our gut has a limited capacity for absorbing most micronutrients, which explained exactly what I was experiencing and seeing in my clinical practice and personal journey. All my observations were just evidence that today's nutritional and biomolecular requirements have far surpassed what anyone could meet just by eating a healthy diet and taking supplements by mouth. There is only so much that our intestine can absorb, and based on my observation, the gut is no longer capable of absorbing enough to meet those biomolecular requirements.

This occurs either because our gut is not that healthy anymore, or our food is not as rich in micronutrients as it used to be, or our requirements are way higher due to modern life's demand and increased levels of stress; it doesn't really matter. The reality is that we need more nutrients to be able to heal the gut and optimize our absorption for at least a period of time. Whether or not this is the optimal route to keep you at the top of your game, that is a philosophical discussion that I will leave for the next book. However, through all these observations, I understood that by bypassing the gut, by using an intravenous route to provide high-quality pharma-graded micronutrients, I was able to overcome all these limitations and get many patients to feel great faster.

Now you might be wondering how fast? Fast, really fast. As fast as the first therapy! That's how fast it is for at least 85 percent of my practice. So yes, I am convinced that PRIME should be incorporated into any patient plan of care to guarantee they get the best results. Exactly as you prepare for a test or a race, the better you prepare, the better you do, and the better outcome you get. The better you prime the body for any activity, the better the body will perform and the better the outcome will be.

Don't you agree that these ideas should be at least entertained as they have potential? In my opinion, we should be looking at this as the next wellness optimization roadmap. At least, that is what it has been for me and my practice. I incorporate it as the first step in any of my protocols and therapeutic strategies to prevent and treat my patients for whatever challenge or condition, no matter what those might be. My philosophy now is "first treat the person, and then treat whatever is left of the diagnosis." This is pretty different from my old days of medical school and hospitalist practice. Simply said, this line of thought revolutionized and transformed not only my medical practice but my belief system forever.

Through this process, I was just using the existing formulas and protocols from the most experienced doctors in the field. This means I was initially just following protocols in a "one-size-fits-all" model. I was even working on creating a compendium of formulas from the most recognized experts in the field. Each formula was assigned or indicated for a specific diagnosis, so my initial catalog was based on the standard, traditional, diagnoses-guided approach that most of my colleagues, even some of the leaders in the field of regenerative and functional medicine, still practice. This is when I met Carlos. I did not know that his case and therapeutic challenges were going to become a main source of inspiration and enlightenment to keep me moving forward.

Carlos was one of the first patients who came to me because he specifically wanted IV micronutrient therapy. He was in his early-forties and had multiple sclerosis. At that point, Carlos was already having difficulties ambulating due to a combination of weakness, spasticity, and balance impairment that forced him to use a cane on bad days. He had progressed to a phase of the disease where there are no longer flares and recoveries, but constant functional and neurological deterioration, known as secondary progressive multiple sclerosis (SPMS). He was following Dr. Perlmutter's Protocol and was very compliant with his diet and plan of care, which included a high dose of IV glutathione.

In fact, he was receiving 2000 milligrams of glutathione IV three times a week by the time he came to me. He told me the dose had been progressively escalated because he was not getting the positive effect from the therapy he used to get during the first few months on the protocols. He insisted he felt great at the beginning, noticing improvement in his level of energy, his leg strength, and coordination. However, he stated that after just a few months on the protocol, he started noticing glutathione was no longer helping him. In fact, he felt like it was making him sick every time he got the shot, getting even worse as the doctor in charge of his care at that time increased the dose.

As I already mentioned, glutathione is one of the major antioxidants produced in our own cells. It's a peptide – tiny compounds of two or more amino acids that can work like hormones. Glutathione is composed largely of three amino acids: glutamine, glycine, and cysteine. Glutathione levels in the body may be reduced by a number of factors, including aging, genetic blueprint, poor nutrition, environmental toxins, and stress. Ascorbic acid or vitamin C is another important antioxidant that is essential for glutathione renewal and positive effects.

Carlos was referred to me by a mutual friend. I noticed he was on a very large dose of glutathione with only oral vitamin C supplementation. He had told me that his vitamin C was checked in his blood, and it registered as almost "0," which he could not understand as his diet was rich in fruits and green vegetables. He also was taking 1000 milligrams of vitamin C twice a day, but he thought I might want to have that checked again.

The scope and accuracy of traditional micronutrient blood testing by current traditional methods is limited because it is based on serum concentration of the different nutrients, which is highly influenced by intake on previous days; it is not necessarily a good reflection of the biomolecular core or body's functional reserve. Therefore, the absence of biochemical evidence of deficiency in those lab results does not imply optimal intracellular levels and might misdirect our efforts toward the wrong nutritional goal.

At the time, I had just started to explore different cutting-edge technology to overcome these challenges. I decided to check his full micronutrient profile using a more functional and dynamic technique than the standard blood test offered by traditional labs. This means that instead of just checking micronutrient levels in blood—in a static and one-time fashion—I used a more functional approach. This functional advanced nutritional testing technology was presented to me at one of the World Anti-Aging Conferences. Their science seemed to be solid, and the doctors using it to guide their patient supplementation plans reported excellent clinical outcomes. The technology was based on isolating the white blood cells (immune system cells) and exposing them to different microenvironments to assess function in the presence and absence of each one of thirty-plus different micronutrients. I ordered Carlos's biomolecular profile. As I suspected, he was severely depleted in not only vitamin C but other micronutrients.

While IV therapy lounges are proliferating throughout the country offering energy boosts and beauty enhancement, there is a hidden risk being ignored by most of the supporters of this growing trend. When IV therapy is given in a "one-size-fits-all" manner without a previous comprehensive medical, biomolecular, genetic assessment, and profiling—and without any monitoring protocol—the short-term risks are minimal, and the benefits seem to be plenty. However, long term, the risks are potentially very significant.

Choosing an IV cocktail by the desired effect, such as beauty or energy or even by a medical diagnosis such as Parkinson's or multiple sclerosis, the formula does not consider your biomolecular core and how this supratherapeutic dose of vitamins and minerals will impact your cellular function. By receiving a supratherapeutic dose of any nutrient such as glutathione, methylcobalamine (MB12), or even vitamin C, you are enhancing and accelerating some pathways that can potentially create long-term imbalances of other micronutrients. As these new pathways are activated, the needs of other nutrients used by the same pathways increases, creating new deficiencies and delaying other pathways that might be essential for your health.

More worrisome than that, these imbalances may impact the expression of your genes, turning on genes that are meant to be off. So yes, we are talking about your genes and gene expression. You might feel great after just one of these infusions, but if you signed up for a weekly or biweekly infusion without any biomolecular monitoring and formula adjustments, you could potentially be getting yourself into a lot of trouble.

Please rethink what you are doing. Biohacking your health is serious business, and it needs to be taken seriously. Just as you get the best advisors to the table before making important decisions for your company or life, you need to do much more than Google it or read an advertisement to make a decision that can impact your health and even your genes at a biomolecular level.

Although all humans are 99.9 percent identical, there are more than three million differences in that tiny 0.1 percent that explains why we all look different, why we can react differently to different drugs, nutrients, and medications. This also explains why our biomolecular core's needs are unique and why you might need certain nutrients more than somebody else. This is the foundation of your biomolecular identity that, in my opinion, will in the future become as important a part of your medical history and therapeutic decisions as your weight, height, age, and gender are today.

As I moved Carlos away from the "one-size-fits-all" approach and started him on a protocol tailored to fill those gaps and meet those unique needs that his biomolecular and genetic profile revealed, he started noticing improvements in his energy level and strength. In time, he turned completely around. I learned that the highest power of IV therapy lies in the possibility of personalizing the formula to the patient's own biomolecular and genetic needs. I also understood that if I was going to bypass the natural nutrition routes, this should be done very carefully and monitored very closely. I decided to dedicate my life to enlightening this field with real scientific and safety protocols.

I had found my purpose. I committed my life to learning and creating more research opportunities to increase awareness of the benefits of incorporating these innovative concepts into the practice of medicine. I founded a company with the main goal to raise resources to promote research to advance the promising field of personalized biomolecular medicine. I also became a real biohacker by eagerly pursuing the latest advancements in the field by aiming to combine the best of science and technology to improve my patient's lives. By recreating micronutrient therapy, I hope we can redesign and reshape the future of medicine; redirecting our effort more towards the basics of what medicine should be; incorporating the concept of bio-individuality into a suffering healthcare system, dying from the foundation up.

Healthcare means we care, and because we care we need to change. It is imperative we reinvigorate the healthcare system from the foundation up by incorporating novel concepts and therapeutic approaches based more on people than numbers. Humanizing the system and individualizing patient care while taking into consideration biomolecular, genetic, epigenetic, emotional, and cultural individuality is what we need to move from a diagnoses-centered model to a patient-centered model. This change would be consistent with the evolution most industries that provide services have experienced in order to meet the new demands modern life has created. We cannot continue practicing under the old model. The healthcare system, medical education curriculum, and even the scientific community and research methods need to be revised openly. It is clear that we are failing as an institution. It is time for us to listen with an open mind and an open heart. I will keep diligently working on it. We all can help.

When Stem Cells Are Upgraded

I was on call during the night shift at Aventura Hospital when I received a call. It was Vanessa, calling from Venezuela. She told me that her husband, Henry, one of our dearest friends, was found confused and unable to speak by a flight attendant. At the same time, my husband received a call from Henry's sister, who lives in Miami, sharing the same story and telling him she was on her way to the airport. The next call I received was from Maximo, my husband. He was already heading to the airport, too. Maximo is a cardiologist. We both knew Henry very well because we went to the same medical school.

We began speculating on what could be happening. We both knew Henry had a condition that increased his risk of blood clotting, and he was taking blood thinners. We thought from the symptoms and his medical history that he was most likely having a stroke. He was forty-two years old at the time. He was going to need to be transferred immediately to a hospital. I got my team ready, as I was on call, and my hospital was a stroke center, in case he could be transferred there. The next call was to tell us the ambulance had transferred him directly to Jackson Memorial Hospital, so everybody met at Jackson then, except me because my shift at the hospital was not yet over.

Henry was received by the stroke team and rushed to the CT scan suite, where it was determined that he was having an ischemic stroke. He was off his blood thinners because he had undergone surgery recently. Next, he was moved to the interventional radiology suite to reopen blood flow to his brain that had been compromised by a massive clot located on his left internal carotid artery. Unfortunately, the next few hours were very dramatic. Despite Henry being placed in the stroke unit and started on blood thinners per standard protocols, clots continued to form and re-occlude the artery again and again.

His initial neurological symptom was expressive aphasia, which means he was unable to articulate his words and write in full sentences. This also explained the first warning sign that his wife noticed. He was texting her a few messages of odd gibberish before she received the call from the airline telling her Henry's flight was returning to Miami, and he was going to be transferred to a hospital. This was just the first sign that the blood flow to his left-brain hemisphere was severely compromised.

As his clotting system continued forming clots on the original spot, his brain function continued deteriorating despite the efforts of the team taking care of him. He was now completely unresponsive, and a full blunt right hemiplegia was added to his neurological exam—this means he was not able to move his right arm and leg because a bigger part of his brain was being compromised by the lack of blood flow. Just a few hours after his arrival at the hospital, his prognosis was guarded. His family were advised to come to the hospital because his risk of dying was high despite being just forty-two years old. That was the situation when I finally finished my night shift and joined my husband at the hospital.

The next few days were a nightmare. Despite everything that was being done to save Henry's brain, the effort seemed useless, and the clots kept reproducing and compromising his left-brain flow. The results were devastating. Although Henry made it through and survived, his left brain was dead. He was unable to speak, write, walk, drive, eat by himself, and his chances of recovery were deemed improbable. Despite that, we all embraced the challenge, thankful he was alive and hoping that due to his young age he could improve and regain part of his neurological function by advanced rehabilitation.

After a few months of intense rehabilitation at Jackson Memorial, he did improve. At the time he was sent home, he was able to ambulate with a splint and speak a few words. He went back to Venezuela to continue his rehab and speech therapy at home.

Unfortunately, his improvement soon hit a plateau. Despite continuing to work hard to accomplish new milestones, his brain seemed unwilling to cooperate. He was left with a full right hemiplegia (right-sided body paralysis) and only able to say fewer than twenty words.

Four years soon passed, and during this time stem cells came into the anti-aging medicine arena. I was fascinated by the science behind them and realized that as important as the biomolecular core was for regular cells, it was also important for stem cells.

Stem cells are like baby cells throughout your body. Because they are in a naive state of development, they have the potential to develop or differentiate into many different types of cells—as such, they are in charge of healing and restoring tissue by creating new tissue. They can stay in a non-dividing and non-specific state for years until the body summons them to repair or grow new tissue by activating them with different chemical signals.

Despite the fact that stem cells are found in almost every tissue, they are difficult to find and isolate. For years we did not know how to activate them into a healing mode, and we thought that stem cells could only differentiate based on their tissue of origin, inducing repair on only specific tissues. We thought that when they were activated, they multiplied and matured into their tissue of origin and there were only a few stem cells in the body—mainly in the bone marrow—that could stay in a state that allowed them to keep the capacity to differentiate into any tissue just like embryonic cells.

Embryonic stem cells can differentiate into any tissue or organ in the process of creating a baby. Most efforts were focused on learning how to find those cells or produce them in the lab, aiming to replicate this amazing healing response by creating new tissues and organs. Unfortunately, it is not that simple, and legal and ethical issues arose, limiting the progress and clinical application of these advancements.

Many scientists redirected their research to look for ways to induce natural healing responses using adult stem cells. They learned that some cells in the bone marrow or even in the fatty tissue could elicit a healing or regenerative response in any tissue. Other scientists started working with perinatal products, such as placenta, cord blood, and amniotic fluid, and discovered that these products could also induce a healing response and recruit and activate adult stem cells to create new tissue. These results were similar to what was seen by the scientists working with bone marrow products and adult fat cells. With time, all these scientists agreed that the active cells that were triggering this healing effect were all the same kind of cells: mesenchymal stem cells (MSC).

When I received Vanessa and Henry's call for help, I had just met a doctor who was working on adipose (fat)-derived stem cells. He was successfully treating patients by isolating MSCs from the patient's fat obtained through minimal liposuction. He had performed many cases with no significant adverse reports; some of them were similar to Henry's case. I talked to him about Henry, and he agreed to incorporate him into his clinical trial.

But I did not want to only have Henry treated with stem cells. I wanted to make sure that he could maximize his chances to get the best response. It made sense to me that if we improved the microenvironment where these cells lived by optimizing Henry's biomolecular core it would be logical to think that these cells could work better. There were also studies that suggested my hypothesis was reasonable, and the doctor was eager to see if that would make any difference because it made so much sense and would not hurt anybody to try.

We delivered the news to Henry and his family, and they all agreed. He came to the States and for the next three months I prepared his biomolecular core for the treatment. First, he underwent bloodwork to assess his biomolecular and genetic makeup. Then we started him on a protocol of personalized IV biomolecular therapy tailored specifically for his individual biomolecular and genetic needs.

Three months went by quickly, and finally the moment of stem cell therapy arrived. Henry stated he was feeling great, and it seemed to all of us that his mindset was also optimal; we all felt optimistic and hopeful about the therapy. The process started with liposuction to get his adipose-derived stem cells. During the cell counting, I was called by the doctor. He was astonished by the findings. Henry's sample was the richest in the number of cells that he had ever seen for somebody of his age and metabolic profile.

The stem cells were prepared and given intravenously to Henry. He tolerated the procedure well, and we were out at a Mexican restaurant just four hours later. The next morning, we met for breakfast, and he was asked what he would like to drink. Henry was bilingual, but since the stroke he had only been able to respond in Spanish. That day he told the girl, "Water, please." He looked at me with an astonished expression. Could this be possible? Could the stem cells already be working?

All I can say is that his progress continues to astonish all of us even now. After four years of a complete plateau, Henry's improvement is more evident every day. Today, Henry is capable of speaking in full sentences, walking independently, and driving. He is also back to teaching medical students and residents and seeing patients. He has become one of those miracles that defy statistics and prove that the best medicine is yet to come.

Henry's great cell count, followed by his amazing response to the therapy, were also the first evidence we found suggesting that optimizing the microenvironment or biomolecular core should become an essential part of stem cell therapy. He was just the first patient of many with similar cellular counts and great outcomes. Physicians who performed the procedures continued reporting consistently enhanced responses to me compared to what they were used to seeing.

These reports added to the reports of others that are working to improve this promising field. Optimizing the biomolecular core is not only important for people's performance and health in general, making them look and feel better, but it can, in fact, make their stem cells work better, which ultimately can make their body and cells biomolecularly and genetically younger!

Potentially these therapies could be used for a more proactive approach, preventing people from getting sick in the first place by optimizing their natural regenerative and healing powers. By activating individuals' own stem cells, we now know we can improve their chances of enjoying what everyone desires: a healthy long life.

Another important lesson I learned was that because these protocols have not been accepted yet as a standard of care in preparation for stem cell therapy, I must work on getting the word out. I cannot hold onto this knowledge. I must find a way to spread it. So, I became a public speaker and started attending stem cell conferences and writing my book.

Unfortunately, the news has not yet spread far enough. Most physicians who are providing stem cells are doing so without preparing their patients' biomolecular core. For me, throwing stem cells into a poor micronutrient environment is like pouring stem cells into a pot of boiling water. Who would do that? Most physicians have been trained that eating well is enough to keep you nutritionally sound—even though that's not accurate.

Now that I have shared this knowledge with you, I hope that you help to spread the word. I hope that you can start to understand the principles of biohacking and practice it responsibly. If you are already interested in health and wellness—which I have to assume you are because you are reading this book—and you are constantly trying new ways to improve your health, whether by using diet and supplements, different exercise modalities and/or meditation, and other similar techniques, you have already experienced biohacking firsthand.

Biohackers combine the best of science and technology to enhance their health and living experience. So please, before spending thousands of dollars on fancy therapies and surgeries, it is important for you to understand that by optimizing your own biomolecular core and your cellular microenvironment, you are most likely enhancing your own healing power, improving your chances of faster recovery and getting better results.

It is also reasonable to think that a clean system would be more beneficial for these cells to exert their healing effect as well. So, cleaning the junk out of your system, helping your body to detoxify better by being a little more careful with your diet, eliminating processed food for a few weeks, and drinking a green juice a day makes sense too. Remember that by optimizing your biomolecular core you also help this natural detox pathway to work better. I hope now you think twice before investing in expensive stem cell therapy or aesthetic procedures and surgeries without preparing your body and improving your biomolecular core first.

RESET, the Inner Chemistry from Disease Progression to Healing

As you know, Henry received fat-derived stem cells or mesenchymal stem cells: MSCs. For many years it has been scientifically recognized that MSCs would be good for creating new fat and connective tissue such as cartilage, but how could they help Henry's brain heal and recover from a severe injury like stroke if those cells were already differentiated? They were not embryonic cells, so they would not by definition be able to repair his brain.

The best way to answer this question is by citing Dr. Arnold Caplan, known in the field as the "the father of the mesenchymal stem cell (MSC)." Based on his work and the work of other great minds in this promising field, we have learned that these more differentiated stem cells orchestrate their healing response not by becoming brain cells themselves, but by producing healing messengers or signals packaged in nanovesicles – tiny nanosized bubbles – called exosomes. It is now widely recognized that the main effect of stem cell therapy has always been its capacity to produce exosomes and elicit a healing response by activating the patient's own stem cells located in the damaged tissue. Even Dr. Caplan urges that we change the name of MSCs to medicinal signaling cells in order to more accurately reflect the fact that these cells, when given as a therapeutic tool, enter the injury site and deliver a healing signal by producing exosomes. In other words, stem cells heal by producing exosomes and resetting the patient's own immune system and stem cells to regenerate and heal, acting more like a medicine delivery system than becoming differentiated cells themselves. It is indeed the patient's own site-specific and tissue-specific resident stem cells that construct the new tissue when stimulated by the exosomes and not the MSCs themselves.

Understanding that the body's inner chemistry is in constant motion, switching from inflammatory/stress mode to healing/recovery mode, regulated by a delicate balance between inflammatory and anti-inflammatory exosomes is key to understand how our body orchestrates the thousands of functions required to keep it healthy. These signals are key to maintaining the delicate balance between healing and inflammation necessary to ensure recovery after any kind of injury and even just the regular recovery that needs to happen every single day of your life.

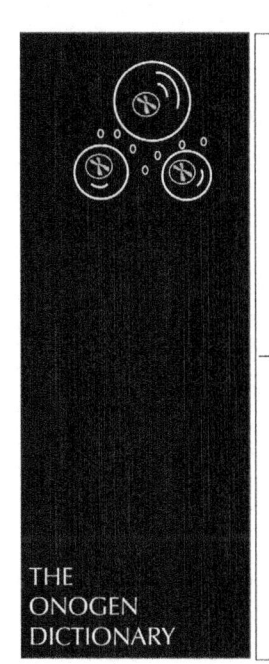

EXOSOMES

NOUN • [ĕksō-sōm]

Signaling shuttles that allow cells to communicate and activate specific genes to orchestrate a specific body's response like immunity, healing, and repair.

THE ONOGEN DICTIONARY

Exosomes are key for cell-to-cell communication. The immune system uses them to activate the body to kill bacteria or viruses and modulate the immune response to balance the inflammatory response, so it does not get out of control and end up harming you. However, as happens with severe infections like sepsis, or with the lung injury seen in COVID-19 and other severe virus infections, sometimes this response can get out of control—the immune system overreacts and causes unwanted harm to the host by creating an undesired chronic inflammatory response. This also happens in patients with autoimmune conditions, where the immune system starts fighting its own body and causes inflammation and organ damage like the joints in rheumatoid arthritis, the intestine in Crohn's disease and ulcerative colitis, or the skin in psoriasis.

Exosomes from MSCs in amniotic fluid seem to play a key role in modulating the immune system, activating a RESET effect, switching the inner chemistry from chronic inflammation to healing and repair, bringing the immune system back in balance. In the particular case of MSCs, their exosomes seem to stimulate healing by activating local stem cells and by modulating the immune system to collaborate with the healing process. These complex effects are explained by the broad selection of specific tissue growth factors, natural anti-inflammatory and immunomodulatory molecules, and even substances with the capacity to turn on or off different genes, enhancing and suppressing specific genes expression, that are packed into these exosomes. These properties make exosomes the key factor triggering the natural healing mechanism seen after infusion of MSCs in patients like Henry, where the tissue involved in the injury—the brain in his case—is considered, traditionally, unable to regenerate or regrow.

Exosomes are produced by cells found in the amniotic fluid during pregnancy known to promote mother and baby well-being and immune synergy and tolerance. Exosomes are also produced by local stem cells after tissue injury or when the cells are cultivated in a lab for the purpose of producing a therapeutic product. Exosomes are found naturally in amniotic fluid and can be isolated by a novel technology developed by Dr. Ian White, who proposed naming these exosomes Cytosomes^{TM}, to differentiate them from exosomes sourced from stem cell culture in a laboratory. In the laboratory, exosomes are found as a supernatant substance in the medium where stem cells are being cultivated and maintained and can be isolated and stored in vials.

Currently, both Cytosomes™ and exosomes are available for use under clinical trials.

I prefer using Cytosomes™, the exosomes extracted naturally from amniotic fluid using Dr. White's technology. First, because amniotic fluid has been used safely in medicine for over 100 years since back in 1910. We all have been exposed to its products and tissue factors while in the womb. And, there is also evidence that the micro-environment within the amniotic fluid at the end of pregnancy is one of the most positive, healing and loving environments, as it has been found to have the highest level in oxytocin found in nature, which probably boost the natural healing and immunomodulatory effect of the exosomes progenitor cells to their highest potential. I hypothesize that this loving boosting effect may explain the higher quality of this product in term of variety and concentration of healing factors when compared to exosomes coming from cell cultivated in the lab.

> "By isolating exosomes from amniotic fluid of full-term healthy pregnancies, we are getting exosomes that carry a broader variety of healing and immunomodulator factors when compared to exosomes coming from other sources."
>
> **—Ian White, PhD**

I even hypothesize, based on abundant literature that supports it, that oxytocin may play a major role in this effectiveness. By obtaining exosomes that come from cells that have been exposed to the most nurturing and loving environment possible, with the highest level of oxytocin in any human sample, we are bringing not only all the natural healing and regenerative effect of these cells to patients, but possibly replicating the state of immune synergy that allows mothers' immune systems to tolerate the baby's presence.

This state of immune synergy could be the answer to aging and the degenerative diseases associated with aging. Even autoimmune diseases could possibly benefit from generating this kind of inner immune synergy. Any strategy or therapy that helps switch from stress/inflammatory mode to recovery/healing mode could bring about the change in the inner environment necessary to trigger this RESET. This concept helps explain how meditation and even touch therapy and love has been reported to trigger healing miracles sporadically throughout human history.

UC Berkeley published one of my favorite studies that demonstrates the effect of oxytocin—the love hormone—on healing and repair processes led by stem cells. The researchers found that by giving oxytocin to old mice they were able to trigger muscle regrowth at a level comparable to young mice—far better than the old control group that didn't get oxytocin. Although still in early stages, these results suggested that increasing levels of oxytocin in the cellular microenvironment appears to rapidly improve muscle regeneration by enhancing muscle stem cell proliferation. This new potential alternative mechanism might explain how love and emotions can impact our biology. Cytosomes™ originate from full-term pregnancy amniotic fluid, when the highest levels of oxytocin are found. As a result, they may hold a higher healing power than any other form of exosomes currently found on the market.

The discovery of exosomes and the chemical signals that activate healing and repair, like oxytocin and other hormones and peptides, have opened new horizons in regenerative medicine. Case reports have been piling up the last two years describing patients who have enjoyed the benefits of all kinds of exosome- and stem-cell-derived products. The first reports were of severe wounds or burns that healed very quickly after only topical application of exosomes. Cases where heart injury after heart attacks and brain injury after stroke have also been reported, demonstrating amazing recoveries after exosome intravenous infusion. Patients with chronic arthritis and severe pain have also reported resolution or significant clinical improvement; even some patients with autoimmune disease have been reported to go into remission or ease the course of their disease, after exosome therapy.

Although this RESET effect has also been achieved through neurobehavioral interventions like meditation and other stress management strategies, exosome data seems very promising. However, we need to understand that these are just preliminary reports of studies that are still ongoing. Despite these promising early observations, their use in clinical practice is still considered experimental. It is reasonably established that exosomes can influence cell behavior. There is a growing amount of legitimate research and excitement about this area, but it is not entirely clear yet if its effects are always beneficial in treating other cells, such as cancer cells. As a result, its use in cancer patients is not recommended.

What captivated my attention since the first day I encountered the science of exosomes is what its potential could be as a tool to induce natural regeneration. Knowing that inflammation and stress are the main culprits of aging, exosomes have the potential to become key therapeutic tools to reset the body to rejuvenation mode, slowing aging and preventing the deleterious effects of time on our body and health.

As my curiosity increased, I began picking the brains of those early researchers and clinicians as to whether any rejuvenation effect had been described by patients who have been treated with exosomes for any other reason. The reports I received suggested that exosome therapeutic applications could positively impact patient longevity and quality of life.

Many patients who received the therapy for different reasons seem to report the same: feeling younger, more vital, and capable of doing things they were not capable of doing before. I know this may sound like sci-fi to you; it did to me, but these reports coming from serious researchers and clinicians have inspired me to incorporate exosomes into my research protocols.

I hope to help with the development of this novel field and accumulate sound evidence to advance toward this vision: a future healthcare system that would be capable of delivering a more preventive and proactive approach to medicine. A healthier approach focused on healthspan and healthy longevity.

PRIME Always Comes Before RESET

As the field continues to evolve; I feel my role is to create more awareness of the importance of optimization of the patient microenvironment before any regenerative therapy. It is well understood that the quality of the micronutrient environment is key for cells to work at their highest potential. Experts have assigned a specific name to the microenvironment where stem cells live—niche. And the niche is considered key to the health and function of stem cells in your body. However, very few physicians in practice implement creating the right microenvironment biomolecularly or emotionally. Research suggests you can chemically change the microenvironment with the production of hormones like oxytocin to optimize healing powers of the stem cell.

My work, as well as the work of other scientists and clinicians, led us to hypothesize that stem cells' integrity, activation, lifespan, and optimal function depend on the nutritional quality of the niche. Based on my observations, the microenvironment balance depends upon the delicate balance of your biomolecular core. My personalized approach to optimizing the biomolecular core seems to be a reasonable tool for improving cell and exosome therapy outcomes. However, people are being treated with regenerative therapies all around the country, and even the world, without preparing this delicate microenvironment before and after to ensure the optimal effect.

Most studies on stem cells link aging with decline of the quality of the nutritional reserve of the niche. The status of your biomolecular reserve is a reflection of the status of your niche's nutritional reserves. This means that when we measure your biomolecular profile, we are uncovering the status of your niche reserve as well, which also means that by optimizing your biomolecular core using a personalized biomolecular formula—your own PRIME—we may enhance the quality of your own stem cells and your self-healing abilities.

The body is in constant renewal. This renewal process depends on the quality of your stem cells. If stem cells are healthy and young, they are capable of multiplying many more times and creating more new cells. As we age, stem cells age with us. As stem cells age, they lose their capacity to function, and they eventually degenerate and die. Studies have linked this process with the deterioration of the micronutrient reserve of the niche. As the micronutrient reserve of the niche deteriorates—mostly explained by multiple factors, such as stress, poor diet, nutrient absorption impairment, use of drugs, alcohol and/or medications, chronic disease, and the aging process in general—healing and tissue regeneration capacity get compromised, accelerating aging and aging-related functional decline, and chronic diseases.

Stem cell research represents for me more clear evidence of how the quality of your biomolecular core can positively or negatively influence your physical and mental performance, vigor, mood, sleep, stress management, skin tightness, and sex drive. But it also influences your ability to naturally self-heal. This regenerative mechanism influences the pace of your body's age clock and your ability to perform day to day in your full power mode.

Moving Your Biomolecular Core from Power-Saver Mode to Full-Power Mode

As we age, small biomolecular deficiencies accumulate, a wearing-out process that is exacerbated by modern lifestyle stress. It slows or even shuts down important biomolecular reactions that are not essential for survival or even to keep you healthy, but they are necessary for your biomolecular core to perform at its highest potential. This is what I call running in power-save mode. As with laptops or mobile phones, when the battery is running down—when your biomolecular core is depleted—some functions of your specific biochemical pathways shut or slow down in an attempt to save resources for life-sustaining essential processes.

As I have mentioned before, when your biomolecular core goes into power-saver mode, your mood goes down just as the brightness of your laptop or smartphone's screen does and your processing speed and capacity to multitask slows down. What happens to you when your biomolecular core is wearing out and your intracellular micronutrient reserves get depleted, your capacity to produce neurotransmitters such as serotonin and dopamine get affected, impacting your mood and outlook on life; it also affects your brain clarity and task-processing speed. Accumulative deficiencies weaken your biomolecular core, preventing you from performing on full power mode. This is reflected in your capacity to enjoy optimal energy, mood, brain clarity, sleep, sex drive, health, longevity, and performance.

Micronutrients, hormones, peptides, exosomes and stem cells are all important factors to define human expression and to help you thrive through life. What I found is that every individual's biomolecular needs are different, and that by meeting those needs, individuals are capable of moving from performing at a standard level to being able to access their natural talents and gifts at their greatest potential. Which, in my opinion, is the kind of medicine we should be aiming for.

But does everyone will need sophisticated and intimidating therapies, such as exosomes or stem cells to get into full power mode? Is the science strong enough to incorporate these innovative therapies broadly in the preventative medicine arena? No, it is not. At least not outside a careful and supervised plan. Besides, most people may just need optimization of their micronutrient environment to replete what has been lost due to stress, aging and day-to-day life. For example, cases like following, whereby just replenishing their biomolecular core they move to a full power mode and are able to achieve their *beyond well* status without using other measures.

John was thirty-eight years old, father of two beautiful girls, and happily married to an amazing and beautiful woman, who happened to be his soulmate. He was a successful entrepreneur in Venezuela. At one time he had a great income and enjoyed the freedom of not living paycheck to paycheck. Then Venezuela started deteriorating politically and financially. He had to move to the States and find a new source of income. He went into a business and was defrauded by his partner. He lost most of his capital and had to reinvent himself. John was forced to move, sell some properties, and become an Uber driver. I have encountered this many times among professional immigrants in Miami during their transition into a new country.

John started working day and night, sleeping very little and neglecting himself while trying to compensate for his loss, sustain his family, and build some capital to create a new business. While in this process, he got sick. It all started when he passed out in his kitchen. His wife and mom were there. It lasted only a few minutes, but it was dramatic. He then began developing different neurological symptoms. First, numbness of his limbs, then weakness of his hands, all associated with severe fatigue and emotional exhaustion.

He underwent an extensive workup at the University of Miami, from advanced blood work to brain and spine MRI. He was also seen by multiple specialists. All the tests were normal, except for an abnormal electromyography, a test used to evaluate electrical activity in response to nerve's stimulation of the muscle. He was also referred to a psychiatrist to help him overcome the hopeless feeling he had developed after all the tests were negative and his deterioration continued. He had days when he could not get out of bed because he could not feel his legs and could not bear his weight. He tried to take what the psychiatrist recommended, but he noticed the side effects of the medication were worse than any benefit he was feeling.

He was referred to me by one of his family members, who happened to be a good friend of mine. I talked to him about the biomolecular core and how I thought this could be the source of many of his symptoms. I wanted to give him a trial. Like many of my younger patients, I suspected he could feel better quickly and become one of those miraculous cases I have seen throughout the years I have implemented these therapies. I knew that by empowering his biomolecular core with nutrients, his hope would return, and his emotions would become his allies instead of his enemies.

That is exactly what happened. I saw him just three times, but after the first therapy his symptoms started subsiding and his strength came back. He was able to slowly incorporate exercise into his routine, and he moved from a regular diet to a cleaner diet—removing processed food, sugar, dairy and gluten, and increasing his intake of fruits and vegetables.

On his last visit he was recharged, back to work, and he stated he felt better than ever. He was working and enjoying taking care of his girls and wife. He said he felt empowered and hopeful. He was also full of gratitude and felt positive about his future, despite the fact his finances were still the same since our first visit three months earlier. He had moved from power saver mode to full power mode.

Call it whatever you want: placebo, psychological recovery, empowerment, personal growth. I have heard them all, and I can tell you that the same effects have been described by other physicians that provide our therapies; even though they are not me, and they might not talk to their patients about their lives and challenges as I do, or they may have a completely different bedside manner. I admit I love to hear my patients' stories, and I love to share with them the tools I have learned throughout the years that have helped me or other patients to overcome challenges, adversity, and hardship.

John was labeled as having depression, and some doctors suggested that his symptoms were a physical manifestation of a psychosomatic mental health condition. However, his electromyography was abnormal. He was referred to a psychiatrist anyway and given a prescription for multiple drugs to calm his anxiety and improve his mood. He took them for a few days and did not like the way they made him feel; he felt even more disconnected and unable to interact with his family than ever and stopped them a few days after starting them.

I commonly see patients that, like John, are assigned mental health labels after laboratories and imaging cannot explain their symptoms. Depression, ADD, anxiety, psychosomatic, mild cognitive impairment, aging-associated functional decline, menopause, andropause, midlife crisis, dementia, and insomnia have all been used to label conditions to match a possible course of therapy with drugs that aim mainly at symptom relief. This is how functional medicine began: a new medical specialty that promises to better address the underlying causes of disease using a systems-oriented approach and engaging both patient and practitioner in a therapeutic partnership. This is a definitive evolution in the practice of medicine that better addresses the healthcare needs of the twenty-first century. New labels popped up with the advent of this new field such as adrenal fatigue, burnout, subclinical hypothyroidism, chronic inflammation, hormone imbalance, mitochondrial dysfunction, and dysbiosis (reduced microbial diversity).

However, despite the fact I am currently using many of the concepts and therapeutic strategies, I do not support all its concepts. I have chosen the ones I believe help me to provide better care to my patients and have left out the ones I disagree with. One of the main problems I have with functional medicine is that it is becoming a new way to prescribe drugs and hormones, following algorithms that do not take into consideration that the most common cause of hormone deficiency and unbalance is secondary to the effect of stress on the individual's biomolecular core. Often the therapy is indicated following a protocol mainly focused on replacing the hormone, leaving out the reason why the hormone imbalance started in the first place.

It seems to me that in modern medicine we easily forget that our body is meant to heal, that each one of our cells holds the miraculous capacity to heal or regenerate itself, or even die if that's necessary to keep the body functioning at its highest capacity. And even in specialties like regenerative medicine, the way therapies are prescribed often ignores the fact that it is our own body that is the protagonist of the healing act. In order to have the best outcome, the main actors, our own cells, need to be provided first with inspiration, nourishment, and nurturing, in the way of personalized biomolecular therapy. In other words, a patient needs to be primed with all those biomolecular factors specifically needed for his or her cells' optimal function. Remember that by optimizing this microenvironment, we are making the cells happier and healthier by changing the inner chemistry of the body.

What do you think you get by making your cells happier and healthier? Yes, a happier and healthier version of *you*! Besides, happy and healthy cells allow you to perform at your very best and to achieve the best results in any endeavor you take on, from a medical procedure to a professional challenge or even a race or marathon.

I'm not saying that medication and medical interventions beside natural biomolecular factors and nutrients are no longer necessary; what I am saying is that if we forget to replenish, protect, and nourish the main player that rules the game, we are unlikely to succeed. Who gives powerful and expensive weapons to weak and untrained soldiers thinking that weapons will win the war? Interventions and medication won't work as well as they could and will likely cause more unbalanced, undesired side effects and harm than they would if your cells were happy and healthy campers.

We need to marry new and traditional medicine by getting them to honor a new concept, in fact, a new foundation. It is a simple concept: optimize healing power by optimizing the microenvironment and biomolecular core as the first line of treatment for any condition. In my opinion, there is no simpler way to do it than by incorporating these novel concepts and the cutting-edge biomolecular technology already available and used by some practitioners like myself. This allows us to finally move on to a new era for personalized, precision, and proactive medicine that will approach each individual based on his or her own bioindividuality, instead of diagnosis or complaints.

Clean Up, Clean Up, Everybody, Everywhere

Increased toxin exposure and stress exposure has been associated with a drastic increase in illness and physical complaints in the last few years. Common chronic degenerative conditions, such as obesity, diabetes, heart disease, migraines, allergies, asthma, digestion disorders, arthritis, autoimmune diseases, and even some types of cancer have all been linked in multiple studies to different toxins and heavy metals accumulation in the body.

Toxin accumulation has also been linked to accelerated aging and aging-related degenerative disease.

Luckily for us, our bodies are very good at getting rid of toxins. Toxins can be produced intrinsically in your body as waste from the natural metabolic pathways or can come from the environment as chemicals found in our air, food, water, and surroundings. Your liver, kidneys, skin, lungs, and intestines all play a role in helping you to detoxify. If these systems are not working effectively to clear toxins from the body, you end up with a toxin buildup.

The amount of toxins that you eliminate or store in your body at any given time is determined by your individual ability to detoxify. Toxins are mostly lipophilic, which means soluble in fat, like any oil. Therefore, most of the environmental pollutants—including persistent organic pollutants

(POPs), pesticides, polychlorinated biphenyls (PCBs), and polybrominated diphenyl ethers (PBDEs)—have been shown to accumulate in fat tissue after exposure. For a while, scientists thought that fat tissue was an inactive storage of fuel, but today fat tissue is recognized as an important endocrine tissue secreting obesity/diabetes-related hormones and immunomodulatory substances as well as a great reservoir of stem cells.

Recent mounting evidence suggests that obesity may represent adverse health consequences of exposure to some of these environmental toxins. These compounds interfere with the body's fat tissue biology and hormone balance. Toxins can break hormone balance by mimicking or counteracting normal hormone function. As a consequence, they are commonly defined as endocrine-disrupting chemicals (EDC). Infants and children are considered a highly susceptible population to EDC exposures; however, evidence suggests that chronic, cumulative exposure during adulthood can be important too. Moreover, exposure to these chemicals seems to play a key role in the development of obesity-related metabolic disorders like diabetes, and even dementia and cardiovascular diseases. While further research is needed to elucidate further the relationship between this exposure and the obesity pandemic and even cancer, it is important to recognize its role as a disruptor of normal cellular function.

After all, your total toxic load is the result of your toxic input minus your toxic output; so, in addition to reducing your overall exposure to toxins (taking less in), you need to make sure your detoxification systems are working well to mobilize and remove toxins. Your individual ability to detoxify determines the amount of toxins that you eliminate or store in your body at any given time. It is also important to understand that by decreasing your toxin input, you are freeing your natural detoxing systems, allowing them to work on previously accumulated toxins and the intrinsic toxins that we all normally produce every day, including hormone waste that, by accumulating, can increase your risk of cancer.

Stress and toxins are undoubtedly connected. The more toxins you accumulate, the more stress your body is subjected to. The first place it shows up is your liver, with elevated liver enzymes and development of what we know today as fatty liver.

Another way that stress compromises your natural detox mechanisms is by altering your microbiome and compromising your intestinal lining. Glutamine, an amino acid found in protein and supplements, is key to the production of glutamate. Glutamate is an excitatory molecule essential for your brain to work optimally while you are awake and under stress. Glutamine requirements increase with stress. However, glutamine is also the main nutrient keeping your intestinal lining healthy. Thus, during stress, your body may compromise your gut health to keep your brain awake, which eventually negatively impacts your nutrient absorption, gut health, microbiome balance, immune system and even your mood. About 90 percent of your serotonin, the neurotransmitter responsible for keeping you positive and happy, is produced in the gut and depends on your gut flora. When these changes occur, the good bacteria and yeast that live in your gut and keep your immune system, digestive tract, and mental health strong, decrease in number. This allows the bad bacteria and yeast to outnumber them, creating imbalance and impacting every single area of your life.

It is also important to understand that when we remove toxins from the body, we need to make sure they are eliminated and not redistributed. Redistribution of toxins can lead to widespread organ dysfunction and damage. In other words, moving toxins that have accumulated in the fat throughout the years and have it deposited in the brain can cause more harm than just leaving the toxin alone in the best tissue to protect you from it, fat.

How can we get rid of toxins and prevent this redistribution from happening?

For toxins—heavy metals and elements, such as mercury, lead, and arsenic, included—to exit fat or any other tissue where they have been deposited, they need to bind to an agent that allows them to dissolve and be carried in the blood to the liver and kidney, where it is processed and eliminated. Chelation agents, such as glutathione, DMSA (dimercaptosuccinic acid), and EDTA (ethylenediaminetetraacetic acid), have been used for years in traditional medicine to do this. They use copper or zinc as cofactors, increasing your bodies' requirements for those elements. They also chelate essential elements such as potassium, calcium, and magnesium, as they are sequestered, transported, and excreted. The increased leaching of essential elements explains many of the symptoms that people experience during chelation therapy that sometimes are attributed to the toxin itself. The change in the biochemical balance itself increases the chance of precipitation and redistribution of the toxins if

CHELATION

NOUN • [ˈkēlāSHən]

The therapeutic elimination of heavy metals and/or minerals and toxins from the body by using molecules with binding capacities.

THE ONOGEN DICTIONARY

it is not addressed correctly. Enhancing natural chelation detoxification pathways, optimizing the biomolecular core, and replenishing the right minerals after appropriate testing and clinical protocols is key. They're needed in order for these therapies to bring all the benefits and prevent undesired complications and side effects.

Detox clean plans, those that make you drink multiple green juices for a few days, can also be detrimental, if your body is not primed correctly with the right minerals, before, during and after. Please understand that by incorporating a large number of natural chelators, such as chlorella, cilantro, watercress, broccoli, and garlic, without understanding the biochemical changes that will happen as a consequence of this intervention, especially if done for long periods of time or very frequently, can compromise your health and biomolecular core balance long term.

When I started prescribing natural detox, I combined juices with compounded powders rich in substances like n-acetyl cysteine (NAC), chlorella, watercress, vitamin C, and B vitamins that naturally enhance the elimination pathways and replenish the reserve of nutrients and minerals most involved in clearing toxins from the body effectively. I've learned the art of detox not only from my own and other experts' and colleagues' successes, but more importantly, by listening to my patients and monitoring their labs and clinical progress. As I no longer have a list of thirty patients to see a day, and I have plenty of time to analyze and try to understand the biomolecular activities behind my patient symptoms, I have developed unique strategies to enhance the detoxification pathways naturally while still keeping that delicate biochemical balance key to successful treatment.

Toxins in the body, and even more importantly, in the nervous system, are best addressed conservatively, with repeated, modest treatments and the use of multiple agents. It is a marathon rather than a sprint. Low initial doses and frequent monitoring with gradual titration, is key to success. With repeated doses the most readily accessed "pools" of toxic elements—mostly in the fat—will be depleted. But there is a re-equilibration that occurs just afterwards that moves the remaining toxic elements to more accessible body compartments than those that have been cleansed. This is more proof that our body is meant to keep us healthy. This is evident in the rebound of levels in the blood following discontinuation of a chelator. Measuring toxins in blood immediately after a detox cycle is just a sign of ignorance and might mislead the physician into giving more therapy at a time when the body just needs a break.

Here is a case that exemplifies how toxins may affect our health. Kim was in her early fifties when she came to me. She is a dedicated and courageous entrepreneur. She was mortified because she felt her brain was no longer working at its full speed, and her mood was down. Kim complained of low energy and stamina, foggy brain and difficulty concentrating. She had seen multiple physicians and specialists. Her hormones were balanced, including her thyroid; her detoxification pathways were checked and optimized; she underwent chelation treatment on multiple occasions. She also stated that her gut and microbiome had been rebalanced with an elimination diet and probiotics. Despite all this effort, Kim still struggled with fatigue and foggy brain and was started on antidepressants by her PCP. She hated the idea but knew that something needed to be done so she could be more functional. She started taking antidepressants while continuing her quest for natural alternatives.

Despite the fact that she had received IV chelation multiple times, no one had ever looked at her biomolecular or micronutrient profile. As we discussed earlier, chelation removes heavy metals but also nutrients and minerals, which can potentially remove necessary micronutrients from your biomolecular core. Kim noticed that sometimes IV vitamin infusions helped her temporarily. But she was not certain because she noticed that the beneficial effects were inconsistent and short-lasting, which was even more frustrating.

Kim noticed that the closest she came to feeling well was after IV infusion. She heard there was a new IV therapy practitioner in Miami Beach who personalized therapies using advanced testing—me. I spent almost two hours on her first visit because her case was very complex. After I gathered all the information and checked all the labs—including extensive genetic profiling she had conducted in the past—I requested her biomolecular and telomere profile. This is performed via a cutting-edge laboratory technology that measures micronutrients and elements functionally instead of in a static fashion, which is how most traditional labs measure them today. I also repeated some basic labs and heavy metals levels.

As I suspected, she had multiple micronutrient deficiencies while her heavy metals profile was not too off. I developed a specific protocol with IV biomolecular therapy specifically formulated to fill the gaps in her profile. We would dedicate a few months to prime her body and recheck heavy metals after. We scheduled therapies every two weeks because her symptoms and labs were consistent with multiple biomolecular core imbalances. I also wanted to give her body and especially her biomolecular core a chance to recover before addressing her heavy metals and hormones. I explained to her that my plan was to replenish her core first and then reassess toxic load and hormones once her core was in better shape and then decide what else was needed.

To make a long story short, she started feeling great almost immediately. She described it as if her brain was awake again, and her energy was consistently available. Her mood improved, and she noticed a remarkable improvement in sleep quality. She felt so great that she started flirting with the idea of getting off the antidepressants.

On the new heavy metal check a few months after the last cycle, mercury was the only one minimally elevated, and we treated it with just a few rounds of chelation therapy, mineral supplementation, and IV glutathione shots. As mentioned before, glutathione is a natural antioxidant, but it is also a key detoxification factor that supports natural detox pathways at multiple and different levels.

The biomolecular deficiencies that I found in Kim are the same I find in most of my patients that describe symptoms such as low energy, fatigue, decreased stamina, foggy brain, memory and focus difficulties, blue mood, anxiety, hot flashes, and decreased sex drive.

As I have accumulated more cases like this, I have come to the conclusion that detox needs to become mainstream. Supported by mounting scientific evidence, it is obvious to me that it is about time to accept that everyone should have some kind of periodic detox plan incorporated into their wellness routine to help them achieve the *beyond well* status that we all deserve to experience in our day-to-day life. I created my own 21-day Detox Plan and Platform. You can find it on this website: https://leafitup.com/.

Beyond Well, a Living Proof

Before we go further, let's recap.

- Deep within your cells, your biomolecular core dictates how fast you age, and how well you look, act, and feel.
- Chronic stress and aging progressively wear off your biomolecular core.
- When your biomolecular core reserve wears off, your day-to-day quality of life, which includes performance, energy, mood, joy, brain clarity, and sex drive, gets compromised, but so does your health, gene expression, and longevity, over the long term, too.
- Missing pieces of this core creates gaps that compromise your natural recovery, healing, anti-inflammatory, and internal regenerative powers.
- Cutting-edge biomolecular and genomic technology available today can help you to identify those gaps.
- Current standard testing is not designed to find these gaps.
- The potential to feel better is within you.
- Biohacking is not a trend—it's self-care 2.0.
- Our healthcare system is overdue for a change.

- By embracing biohacking, we are supporting the shift of our current outdated medical model towards a more participative, equalitarian, empathic, and inclusive healthcare system.
- Do not settle for being well, strive for being *beyond well*— a status of health and well-being where you live, operate, perform, look, and feel way beyond what you think "at your best" is .
- Do not just age! Age *beyond well*, growing and thriving into the healthiest, happiest, and best version of yourself.
- Your health is your wealth. Prioritizing in your own health and investing in healthy longevity is one the best contribution you can make to your future self.

CHAPTER 4

Genes Are Not Your Destiny

If you haven't heard of this concept before, you might be amazed, just as I was when I heard it for the first time. I was under the impression, after many years of medical school, that genes were static—like a death sentence. So, it is better not to know what you have if you cannot change it. That's what I used to think. All these misconceptions have changed in the last few years as we have learned more about genes and how gene expression is modulated.

Every cell in your body contains the genetic code that makes you "YOU." DNA carries your genetic instructions for the development, growth, reproduction, functioning and longevity of all life. The code is written so it can't be changed. However, there are parts of the code that are OFF, that can remain OFF for the rest of your life, or can turn ON depending on environmental factors; diet, exercise, stress, love and environmental toxins can all modulate the gene expression in a positive or negative way.

I know it sounds complicated, but please don't quit yet. What I am describing is very empowering and can even be life-changing. What I am trying to explain here is that everyone has genetic potential. If you do the right things—eat right, exercising and training your brain to have a positive outlook on life, keeping your biomolecular core in good shape—you can potentially unleash all the good in your genes and achieve BEYOND WELL. If you do the wrong things: don't dedicate time to develop your personal formula to manage stress, stay healthy, and ignore your unique biomolecular core's needs, you may unleash negative genes that you'd rather stay dormant during your lifespan.

Although this is a young science, there are many factors that we already understand well enough to start utilizing for our own and our children's and children's children benefit.

Defying Your Genes

When I was three years old my mom was told I was pretty much broken. I had multiple congenital deformities in my spine. Doctors told her they needed to rule out kidney and heart malformations as well, as often these kinds of malformations are linked to spinal malformations.

Of course, for my mom it was very hard to take. How could I look perfect and be that broken? Thankfully, the kidney and heart tests came back okay, but she was told that as I grew, I was probably going to need multiple surgeries for my back or I would most likely look like the Hunchback of Notre Dame.

Literally. I'm not trying to be overly dramatic: this was exactly what she was told.

Thankfully, my uncle was a wise man who also happened to be an orthopedist, whose wisdom and common sense helped my mom overcome this difficult time. My uncle told my mom that if she got me into a good exercise regimen including swimming and ballet, we could perhaps defeat this prediction.

We embarked on this journey, and I practiced ballet and swam for many years. I never required surgery and ended up developing a muscular, well-balanced back. These days my friends and family compliment me, saying I have a sexy back. I owe it to my uncle and my mom's defiant response to the challenge.

This was a defining event for my mom and our relationship. I think this gave my mom the idea that our destiny was really in our hands, and with hard work and faith, even genes could change. Maybe she transferred this belief to me. Perhaps I owe my rebel spirit to the way this event transformed my mom and her belief system, which obviously influenced mine and manifested in many of my decision-making processes through life—like when I learned I was pregnant for the first time.

I had just finished my residency and gotten married a few months before. My husband and I were already in the United States taking our medical boards and getting ready to apply to residency programs and getting started with training in the United States. I was in my late twenties, and my first response to pregnancy was to go online and check on everything that had been published that could help my baby to be as healthy and happy as he could be.

One of my challenges was that both of us, my husband and I, had asthma during childhood. *Asthma* runs strongly in families and is about half due to *genetic* susceptibility and about half due to environmental factors. This meant that per statistics our offspring would have a high chance of suffering the same destiny.

I made it my mission to find literature that could help me develop a strategy to defy this forecast and give our children a better chance for a sunny and clear childhood. A review article suggested that moms who followed a hypoallergenic diet during pregnancy decreased their offspring's risk of having asthma during their childhood. I embarked on the journey of pregnancy, experimenting with a hypoallergenic diet. By that time, I was no longer vegan, but I was eating a healthy diet rich in vegetables and dairy. So, my major challenge was to get dairy (a common allergen) out of my diet, being a cheese lover. My addiction to cheese was so bad that I had to have cheese at every freaking meal: breakfast, lunch, snack and dinner. Yes, I was a cheese addict.

But my love for my baby was more than my love of cheese, so I quit cheese and dairy, and the first thing I noticed was that my eternal rhinitis and sinus congestion disappeared, and my eyes stopped itching every morning. Besides my sinus and eye problem going away, the result of all this was two babies who are now healthy teenagers who have never had asthma or bronchial problems.

That doesn't mean that the genes are not there—they are there for sure—but they are not expressing, they are OFF, probably in part explained by my commitment to the hypoallergenic diet during pregnancy followed by the late introduction of dairy in my children's life. I breastfed for a year, only introducing table food around six months of age and dairy after two years of age. Even then, they still were exposed to dairy sporadically instead of the typical three glasses of milk recommended by the authorities in the field.

This decision was a little disturbing to my pediatrician, but we both decided to ignore it. In my case, I was convinced that the standard was not always right. For him, perhaps, because my kids were growing well, and their mom, my younger self, was persistent about these crazy ideas. So, just as my mom worked to defy my genetic prediction, I did too with my children. And a surprise to many, despite the lack of dairy, we all survived, including the mortified and patient pediatrician whom I love to this day.

This is how I learned the concept of epigenetics firsthand in my life. By the time I was in medical school and learned all about DNA, my rational vision was that genes were static—even though intuitively I knew this was not right. I did not put it together until now while writing this book. For me, at that time, genes were your destiny, and there was nothing you could do to defeat them.

Epigenetics: A New Frontier in Preventive Medicine and Human Enhancement

Epigenetics is the study of changes in organisms caused by modification of gene expression rather than alteration of the genetic code itself. There are specific molecules along the DNA, such as methyl groups—a carbon atom and three hydrogen atoms—that can act as a switch to turn genes *on* or *off* depending on certain environmental factors.

The studies I read to embark on a hypoallergenic diet during my pregnancy, as well as other studies, provide evidence that prenatal and early postnatal environmental factors influence the child's risk of developing various chronic diseases and behavioral disorders throughout their lifetime.

Think of a caterpillar and a butterfly. Think of the process of human development from infancy to the growth and changes occurring through childhood and puberty in response to hormones and environmental stress. Think of all that, and you'll understand that epigenetics is what happens when genes are actually in action.

In all of these processes, genes are the same in terms of their structure and code, but functionally they express and act differently.

Nessa Carey, PhD and author of *The Epigenetics Revolution and Junk DNA*, compares genes to a script for a play rather than a fixed template. The same script can produce different productions of the same play.

New and ongoing research is continuously uncovering the role of epigenetics in a variety of human disorders and fatal diseases. Unfortunately, most studies are mostly focused on disease diagnosis and treatment. Its implications for human enhancement and disease prevention are still lacking.

As we learn more about these epigenetics mechanisms, it has become clearer that epigenetic effects occur not just in the womb. Even though our genes seem to be more stable during adulthood, numerous studies show how different lifestyle choices and environmental exposures in a very short period can alter DNA expression. This has implications for how to improve health on an individual level for a variety of conditions, from cardiovascular disease, hypertension, diabetes, autoimmune disease, and even cancer.

Today we know that certain biomolecular imbalances, micronutrient deficiencies, environmental toxins, and even chronic stress, negativity, strained relationships, and low self-esteem can deeply affect your gene expression.

However, it's also well-known that a healthy diet, optimal quality of sleep, smart exercise, and stress management can not only positively impact gene expression but can reverse previous epigenetic changes. So, epigenetic changes can occur over the full course of a human lifespan, and previous epigenetic changes can be reversed. The switches can be turned off and on.

How did this happen? How do outside behavior and environmental factors impact gene expression? And how can these changes also impact your lifespan as well as your chance of a healthy and happy life through those extra years? These are questions that are being answered by progress in the field of epigenetics.

Currently, one of the most broadly studied and well-characterized epigenetic modifications is known to occur through DNA methylation, which I cover in the next section. DNA methylation involves very small chemical modifications (usually the addition of a tiny methyl group to one base of DNA) turning genes *on* or *off*.

I like to compare the methylation process to unlocking a door, so a key. In this case, the methyl groups are the only ones that can regulate whether the door is opened or closed, allowing your genes to be expressed or not.

Methylation: The Key to Optimal Health

Methylation is a key biochemical process by which methyl groups are added to different molecules: a process that is essential for the proper function of almost all of your body's systems. Methyl groups are a "key essential" to lock and unlock the doors or gates that regulate the most important functions of your body. So, you need just the right number of keys—not too many, not too few. This locking-unlocking process occurs billions of times

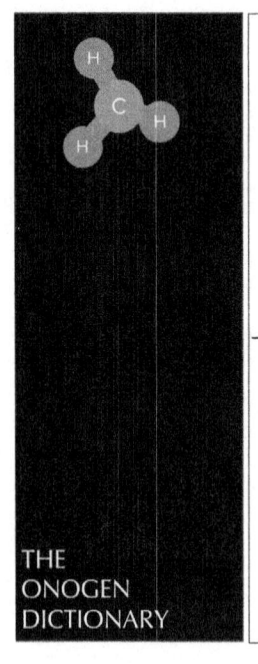

METHYLATION

NOUN • [meth-uh-ley-shuhn]

A biochemical process by which methyl groups are added to different molecules: a process that is essential for the proper function of most of the body's systems.

THE
ONOGEN
DICTIONARY

every second and even more times when you are more active or under stress. It regulates your DNA repair on a daily basis and your vitamins' activation, making them available to your cells to use for your benefit; it helps balance your hormones and get rid of environmental toxins by recycling molecules needed for detoxification; it also controls homocysteine (an unhealthy compound that can promote inflammation, bone loss, and blood vessel damage). Optimal methylation is also key to maintaining a positive mood by regulating neurotransmitter production, like serotonin and dopamine, and keeps immune response and inflammation in check.

These keys—methyl donors—play a very significant role in our body's ability to utilize nutrients and turn genes *on* and *off*. This means that methylation can change the activity of a DNA segment without changing the sequence. Our understanding of these genetic expression modulation mechanisms has turned what we have long held true about biological destiny upside down. This intriguing finding means that your genetic heritage is not the primary determinant of your health, disease risk, or longevity.

Every time your body goes through periods of increased demand, stress, or exposure to environmental toxins, different medications, alcohol, or drugs, you need more keys to cleanse your system and keep up with baseline gene maintenance, immune system function, vitamin activation, and hormone metabolism. If there are not enough keys, some of these processes become compromised. And so do your physical, mental, and even spiritual—at least I believe this last one gets affected—performance and eventually your health.

Because the keys in your system are scarce during this demand-increased period, you may feel signs of system malfunction, such as lack of energy, increased brain fog, sleep disturbances, and mood swings. If these signs are ignored, the scarcity of keys can end up affecting essential organs and systems, causing events that may create imbalances that trigger processes that end up manifesting as chronic diseases. These run the gamut, including cardiovascular disease, diabetes, thyroid disease, neurotransmitter imbalances, inflammation, immune dysfunction leading to autoimmunity, chronic infection and cancer, neurodegenerative disorders, psychiatric disorders, and premature aging.

In order to keep your methylation at optimal function and reduce the deleterious effects of methylation defects, you need to ensure that you are getting enough keys or methyl factors. Increasing the amount of methyl-related nutrients in your diet is a great way to start. It is also important to understand how well your body is processing and utilizing these keys, which you can find out with very simple bloodwork tests, such as having your doctor check your homocysteine levels and MTHFR gene status.

Where Do I Get These Keys From?

The keys, the methyl groups, can directly be delivered by dietary methyl donors including methionine, folate, betaine-choline, B vitamins, and SAMe (S-Adenosyl-Methionine). It is very important when choosing your supplements to read the label and make sure that the B vitamins and folate come in their active, methylated form. This means that you want a multivitamin that has methylfolate and methylcobalamin instead of just folic acid and cyanocobalamin (B12).

Finding foods that are good sources of methyl donors isn't difficult if you are mindful of your choices and eat a lot of vegetables, beans, and unprocessed food. Although eating food rich in these keys is helpful to provide more keys to your body and a certain way to stress-proof yourself, in my own experience diet alone is not enough to supply the needed amount of keys to excel in our modern, demanding society. However, there is a way for you to monitor how you are doing, by checking your blood homocysteine levels every six to twelve months.

In my practice, I correct the levels as needed by adjusting each individual's personalized, intravenous biomolecular formula. I use the formula to reinforce what they are doing with their diet because I have learned that the chance of fully meeting your personal requirement just by eating food rich in methyl donors is very low, especially in those with a highly demanding lifestyle!

However, never forget that what you eat is still key to your health, and any oral or parenteral, intramuscular, or intravenous supplements should be just that, supplemental to your diet. This means eating foods rich in methyl factors should be as important to you as supplementing with methyl donors.

Here are some examples of food and nutrients to enhance your methylation pathways:

- **Folate:** chickpeas, lentils, pinto beans, leafy greens (e.g., spinach, kale, collards, mustard greens, bok choy), strawberries, and citrus (e.g., grapefruit, oranges, lemons)
- **Vitamin B6:** grass-fed beef, pistachios, pinto beans, avocado, blackstrap molasses, tuna, sunflower seeds, sesame seeds
- **Vitamin B12:** fish, organic meats, seaweed (laver and nori), eggs
- **Methionine:** Brazil nuts are a super source, while other excellent-to-good sources include sesame seeds, roasted soybeans, parmesan cheese, tuna, eggs, and white beans
- **Choline** (which oxidizes to a methyl called betaine): beets, brussels sprouts, broccoli, liver, eggs, raw cauliflower, cooked beet greens, cooked asparagus
- **DMG** (Dimethylglycine): beans, brown rice, pumpkin seeds
- **DMAE** (Dimethylamine): anchovies, salmon, sardines
- **SAMe** (pronounced Sammy): there are no direct food sources of SAMe; however, it is a compound made from methionine, so it is acquired indirectly. There are supplements of SAMe on the market. They are known for their mood and immune modulation properties and to promote joint health

A good balance of methyl donor foods as part of a natural foods diet can help promote and support optimal methylation. In addition, getting a sufficient amount of zinc and magnesium, which are also essential cofactors on the methylation pathways, is as important to make yourself stress-proof and to optimize your body and mind performance.

MTHFR aka "The Mother F...er" Gene

Roughly 40 to 50 percent of people have mutations in the gene that codes for the production of a key enzyme known as the MTHFR (methylenetetrahydrofolate reductase enzyme). This enzyme is crucial to the proper function of the methylation pathway and the production of methyl donors. The high frequency of mutation in the gene coding for this crucial enzyme and the impact that this mutation potentially can have on our health is the main reason that explains why the enzyme-gene acronym is also comically known as the "Mother F...er." It's a name that I used to make sure my patients don't forget the name of the enzyme if they have any of the mutations in this gene. It is also good to be able to deliver this kind of news with a sense of humor so people can laugh about it. After all, laughing about your imperfections is usually the first step to overcoming them. Besides, it is not such a big deal. It is just a difference that determines that the requirement of keys, methyl groups on these individuals, is higher than the general population. It is just one more characteristic that I use to create those unique personalized formulas for my patients.

People can have either one or two defects, known in genetics as SNPs (single nucleotide polymorphisms, pronounced "snips"), or can have neither on the MTHFR gene. These defects more often occur at two areas, also called variants, C677T and A1289C. We all carry two copies of the gene, and we inherit a single copy from each of our parents. One would hope that both copies inherited would be normal, but, more often than not, there are defects that occur and are passed down from parent to child. The number and type of defects impact the expression of the gene and the production of the enzyme differently, causing disruption of pathways and affecting cell function at different proportions.

The statistics for each specific variant are:

- C677T. Approximately 30 to 40 percent of the American population may have a mutation at gene position C677T. Twenty-five percent of people of Hispanic descent and 10 to 15 percent of Caucasian descent are homozygous (have two mutations) for this variant.
- A1298C. Around 20 percent of the American population may have a homozygous mutation at gene position A1298C.
- It's also possible to acquire both C677T and A1298C mutations (one copy of each).

People with just one mutated gene (heterozygous) may not see the negative effect unless they are under very stressful circumstances, either physical or emotional. Examples of physical situations that can increase your requirements are: poor diet, biomolecular deficiencies, strenuous exercise activity, exposure to cigarettes, alcohol, drugs, medication, too much caffeine (more than two coffees or caffeine beverages a day), environmental toxins or heavy metals, chronic pain, or inflammation. Examples of emotional situations are chronic stress, strained relationship with inner self or others, depression, negativity, and low professional satisfaction. People with a double mutation (homozygous) usually need daily methyl donor support in the form of supplements to stay healthy and prevent metabolic disruptions that could compromise their health in multiple areas.

There are plenty of methyl support supplements on the market, such as SAMe and methylated folate and B vitamins. I usually prefer to prescribe SAMe by mouth associated with no more than 800 mcg of methylenetetrahydrofolate and 1000 mcg of methylcobalamin.

The keys, or methyl factors, are also essential for the production of new DNA and RNA in our cells. As cells die and need to be replaced (literally millions of cells every minute), DNA and RNA need to be produced. If the process is slowed down, new cell production cannot keep up with cell death (apoptosis) and aging, which can accelerate the aging processes. Mutations or defects in cellular regeneration and DNA formation can also result in aberrant creation, increased mutations, and DNA repair failure, which may result from the lack of enough methyl factors, usually expressed as aging-related disease or even cancer, hormone imbalances, infertility, and autoimmunity.

The systems most affected by DNA replication disruption associated with insufficient key methyl factors are the bone marrow's erythrocytes and lymphocytes, as well as neural tissues, the digestive system, skin, hair follicles, and nails. All are the most rapidly growing and dividing cells of our bodies. This explains why stress and episodes of high demand usually first affect your immune system, increasing the risk for catching a cold and flares of chronic viral conditions like cold sores, herpes, or shingles. It also explains why people tend to develop digestive issues, hair loss, and brittle nails when under stress. The effect of stress on the skin is also evident as eczema, dandruff, and even psoriasis flares and vitiligo. High levels of stress have been linked as well to accelerated skin aging, with more wrinkling and loss of turgidity and glow.

The impact on the brain and mood are also to be considered based on the MTHFR genotype. These key factors are also critical for the production of essential neurotransmitters. Neurotransmitters are those chemicals that allow our brain and neurons to communicate and translate into feeling happy, active, focused, or sleeping. For example, dopamine, oxytocin, *serotonin*, and endorphins all play a role in how you experience happiness. Therefore, deficiency of methyl factors has been associated with clinical depression. Furthermore, SAMe supplements have been shown in multiple studies to naturally treat depression. These studies suggest SAMe as an effective nutritional and natural alternative to treat depression. In my opinion, SAMe is one of the safest, most well-studied, and most effective natural remedies for depression symptoms. I usually utilize it with my patients with mild symptoms—especially those with MTHFR mutations—in the presence of elevated levels of homocysteine in their blood. Although I have not found published research that supports this personal approach, I have implemented and added it to my protocol; my common sense prevails here, and it has been working for my patients and even myself. Yes, I am carrier, heterozygous on the C677T variant, so I take it as well.

It is very important to understand that if you have symptoms of depression, you should seek medical attention and discuss with your physician any changes in your regimen before trying any new supplement, even SAMe, as you can create undesired interactions and end up having more problems.

Most traditional physicians check folate and B12 levels in the blood as part of multiple test profiles for fatigue, memory loss, and anemia. However, today we know that the blood levels of these nutrients are not really the best reflection of the intracellular values for them because the blood levels are directly related to their intake but may not reflect the intracellular status of the same nutrient. Today's processed foods are enriched with folates and B vitamins, and despite your fasting status, if you have eaten food enriched with vitamins prior to blood being drawn, your levels of vitamins in your blood are a better reflection of what you have been eating rather than what you really need. Knowing the MTHFR genetic status is also helpful, but this tells us only if the individual has a predisposition to folate and B12 deficiency, which does not necessarily mean that the individual is deficient at that moment. This is partially why this area of medicine lags behind—because the accuracy of the technology available to measure nutrients has been limited for many years.

The best way to track methylation is by checking and monitoring homocysteine, a simple and widely used blood test, available in any standard laboratory.

Elevated homocysteine level is a reliable marker for your own methylation status and is one of the values that I monitor in my patients every six months to adjust their personal formula aiming to keep their methylation pathways working properly. Elevated homocysteine is recognized as an independent risk factor for cardiovascular disease. High homocysteine has also been linked to other problems, including osteoporosis, birth defects, macular degeneration, and certain types of cancer. In addition, some evidence suggests that people with elevated homocysteine levels have twice the normal risk of developing cognitive impairment in the form of Alzheimer's dementia. High homocysteine is also associated with low levels of vitamin B6, B12, folate, and renal disease.

Despite an elevated plasma level of homocysteine long known as an independent predictor of cardiovascular disease, the American Heart Association (AHA) guidelines do not include this test as part of the standard test for cardiovascular risk stratification. This is the reason your doctors probably haven't checked your levels. Most mainstream doctors still do not accept elevated homocysteine as a modifiable risk factor compared to the classic lipid-related risk factors for heart attack and stroke, high LDL, triglycerides, and low HDL.

Do you want to know the reason why? Because the research that supports the need for treating high cholesterol is supported by big pharma. Somebody is making money, and the studies and research get funded with the ultimate goal of making a profit. I'm not saying that they don't care about the benefits that humanity gets by looking for new drugs and fancy therapeutic tools, but the reality is, nobody makes a massive amount of money by giving patients vitamins, so nobody funds this kind of research.

I used to be blinded to these facts until I started thinking more about it and listening to other experts' opinions on the subject. I am not trying to make a political statement here, or getting into areas outside of my expertise, I am just describing a fact I have encountered throughout my year of practicing medicine in this current economic model. As any model has strengths and weaknesses, this is one of those weaknesses that I feel is affecting us. As a result, a significant and cost-effective preventative strategy is ignored for close to fifty years because nobody wants to invest in it.

This is one of the weaknesses I want to help overcome. And the first way to do it is by creating awareness to the fact that this weakness exists, and we all have to work together to overcome it.

In the meantime, in the absence of a clear mechanism linking homocysteine to cardiovascular disease, the ongoing debate continues, and thousands of patients miss the opportunity to improve their risk profile with a simple, affordable, effective, and harmless intervention. The simple supplementation with methyl donors also brings benefits in other areas of health besides cardiovascular health, including brain, bone, immunity, gastrointestinal, joint, and genes benefits.

I want to empower you to ask your provider to check your homocysteine levels. If he or she tells you it is not necessary, ask him/her to read this chapter, or have them contact us through our website: https://onogen.com/contact-us/. Help me to wake them up and create more awareness.

As I mentioned previously, there is evidence connecting cancer with the methylation pathway. What we have learned in the last few years is that in the presence of either excess or deficiency of methyl donors, your genes may experience significant modulation. Your DNA repair mechanism may become partially impaired, with over- or under-methylation of particular genes that turn *on* and *off* tumor growth, known as tumor suppressor genes.

A well-balanced methylation status is key to keeping your genes expressing optimally. This means that by monitoring and optimizing homocysteine levels we may be able to suppress or inactivate certain areas of our genes that can cause a rise in cancer expression. The methylation-cancer connection is also linked to the effect of methylation on the detoxification and metabolism of hormones. Some estrogens can cause cancers, and methylation of estrogen reduces this effect. Methylation also plays a role in our immune system to identify cancer cells, and, in particular, NKT (natural killer T-cells) cells, to recognize and destroy cancer and potential precancer cells. Therefore, people with poor methylation function may be more susceptible to cancers.

Methylation also plays a role in controlling and modulating the immune system response against your own tissues, so methylation problems have been linked to different autoimmunity manifestations.

Methylation is also critical to the process of removing toxins and the production of glutathione. As you now know, glutathione is an antioxidant that plays a key role in different detoxification pathways. These properties also make glutathione a key player in the immune response helping to control inflammation and cellular aging. As with glutathione, methylation and methyl donors tend to decrease with age. Imbalances of the methylation pathway impact the speed at which we age. Maintenance of our body's ability to methylate will stave off degenerative diseases of organs associated with the aging process.

While DNA methylation is one of the most broadly studied and well-characterized epigenetic modifications and has been associated with cellular aging and a proposed mechanism to calculate biological age, the discovery of telomeres and its role in aging has pushed this science forward and has become the most recognized predictive biomarker of health and longevity.

CHAPTER 5

Telomeres, DNA, and Immunity: Turning Back Your Body Clock

The significance of telomeres in health and aging came to public attention when Elizabeth H. Blackburn, Carol W. Greider, and Jack W. Szostak were awarded the Nobel Prize in Physiology and Medicine in 2009 for their discovery of "how chromosomes are protected by telomeres and the enzyme telomerase." Since then, significant research has shown that keeping your telomeres—the DNA caps at the end of your chromosomes that protect your genetic data—in optimal condition, can protect you from chronic diseases, and physiological and functional deterioration associated with aging.

Just like the plastic tip on the shoelace, telomeres are the end caps that protect our chromosomes and keep the DNA from unraveling. The longer the plastic tips at the ends of the shoelaces, the less likely they will fray. Therefore, the longer your telomeres are, the more protected your chromosomes are and the better your cellular forecast becomes for a healthier

> **THE ONOGEN DICTIONARY**
>
> CHROMOSOME (DNA)
> TELOMERE
>
> ## TELOMERES
>
> NOUN • [tēləmi(ə)r]
>
> end protective caps of your chromosomes that hold the power of healthy and sexy longevity

and longer life experience. Unfortunately, every time your cells replicate during the aging process, a part of your telomere fades away. When they become too short, the cell throws itself into senescent or suicidal mode, which means cells stop replicating and functioning. This results in aging-associated deterioration, as well as chronic diseases that affect your quality of life.

The presence of excessive immune-senescent cells or dying immune cells has been found to actively compromise the immune system capacity to modulate inflammation, causing this state of low, chronic inflammation called inflammaging. Inflammation causes immune dysfunction, which leads to more immunosenescence, and that feeds right back into inflammaging. Which becomes a never-ending loop.

We Age Because Our Immune System Ages

Immune cells and stem cells are key signaling systems in charge of healing processes, fighting infection and cancer, modulating inflammation, and pacing aging. While young cell signals activate healing, recovery, and regeneration, exhausted senescent cells, those whose telomeres have shortened and lost their ability to divide, on the other hand, produce pro-inflammatory signaling, triggering aging, and organ function decline and deterioration.

Aging signs start appearing when the aging signals overcome the healing signals, causing everything from graying hair to inflammaging, immunosenescence, hormone imbalances, and aging-related decline and diseases.

The body's inner chemistry is constantly swinging between inflammaging and healing, survival and recovery mode.

As our biological clock ticks, more senescent cells accumulate in every organ. It is calculated that by the chronological age of sixty, the inflammaging signaling start prevailing over the repair signaling, due to the accumulation of these dysfunctional cells, breaking the delicate balance that allows us to repair, heal, and thrive effectively throughout our younger years. Although this phenomenon start developing in our forties, it really expedites after the age of sixty, as seen on the drop of different immune cell lines, like the CD8 Killer and CD4 Helper immune cells, mainly in charge of tissue healing, immune system regulation, viral and cancer immune defense, and the age-related deterioration of the thymus composition. This causes aging-related immunity and organ function decline, contributing to the development of chronic degenerative diseases, such as heart disease, atherosclerosis, diabetes, dementia, arthritis, and cancer.

Therefore, telomere length and the immune signaling system are key regulators not only for your lifespan but also the quality of life of those years you'll live, or healthspan.

From Lifespan to Healthspan: New Goals, New Era

Despite the average lifespan having increased in America over the last twenty years, the quality of life of those last years gained does not seem to be following the same trend.

Chronic illness and functional decline start picking up after the age of sixty for most Americans. Given that lifespan is seventy-nine in the United States, this means that most people live up to 20 percent of their lives burdened with aging-associated illness and disabilities.

Focusing on longevity should not be our main goal in medicine. Our main goal should be cultivating strategies to optimize the quality of those

LIFESPAN

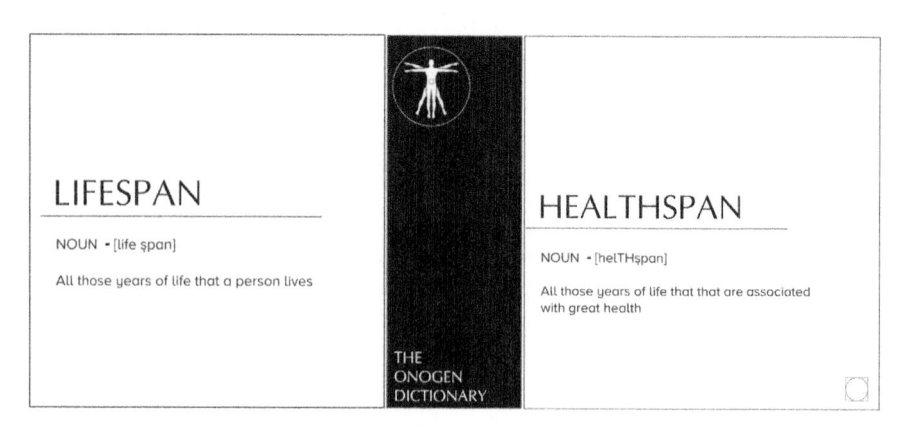

NOUN • [līf spən]

All those years of life that a person lives

HEALTHSPAN

NOUN • [helTHspən]

All those years of life that that are associated with great health

THE ONOGEN DICTIONARY

years, making sure that medicine not only helps people to live longer but better. This is how the concept of healthspan was born.

Healthspan is defined as those years of life that are associated with great health. It means that you are adding years of great health instead of just adding years to your life. Isn't this what everyone wants?

It is not that easy. There is not yet a magic pill to bring you this wonderful benefit. But there is enough knowledge and technology to allow you to create a plan that could increase your chances of living younger longer, promoting your healthspan. The first step is making this one of your priorities. After all, your quality of life and the years you add to your life with great health are probably the biggest asset you can create.

But you need to understand that what most people in America are doing to improve their chance of a long and healthy life is just not enough. If your idea of taking care of yourself is just going to your doctor for an executive physical once a year and getting regular blood work, including lipid profile, mammogram, and Pap smear—if you are a woman above forty years old—and prostate-specific antigen (PSA) if you are a man above forty years old—and a colonoscopy after fifty for both genders, you are doing something important, but it won't be enough. These are tools that help extend your life by promoting early diagnosis and treatment of the most common age-related health problems. These tools are screening strategies. You already know from reading the previous chapters of this book that there is more to offer in terms of prevention than just these strategies.

As we have discussed, a biomolecular core in full power mode and optimal methylation are essential factors to maintain genetic integrity and stability of your DNA. So are your telomeres.

It is time to start taking our internal micronutrient environment and biomolecular core integrity seriously. Understand that most of the age-related problems we see in medicine—including problems as common as weight gain, hormone imbalances, and memory loss and functional decline—are many times just an alarming sign of the biomolecular core reserve wearing off. By understanding this, we are able to redefine the future of medicine, moving from the current reactive approach to a real preventive approach.

There are cutting-edge medical diagnostics that are available today. This includes things such as advanced micronutrient and biomolecular profiling in combination with genetic and telomere-length analysis. I have incorporated them into my practice. Unfortunately, most insurance companies do not cover this kind of blood work. Therefore, we can provide this approach only to those privileged people who are able to afford the cost of this advanced technology. Hopefully, this will change soon, as in my opinion, this testing can potentially provide you with more comprehensive insights into your health and aging pattern than many standard testing strategies covered by most insurance companies.

For my part, I am determined to continue creating research opportunities to obtain the necessary data to meet the requirements needed to validate these strategies as an essential part of any individual medical evaluation. That is to say, to make them as common as blood pressure measurement, weight and temperature. I am already using and gathering data that support this approach in my medical practice, creating unique, personalized therapies that target my patients' individual cellular needs at a molecular level.

By optimizing your biomolecular profile, you not only improve your chance of living longer with greater quality health, but you may improve your cellular function and enhance your energy level, stamina, performance, brain clarity, mood, sleep, and sex drive. This will impact every area of your lifestyle and improve your chance of achieving your highest potential.

I try to explain this to all my patients. It is a great way to open a space for discussion about other strategies that are also conducive to the same benefits that I recommend incorporating in their lifestyle. Things like eating more plants, good protein, and fats, fasting, exercising regularly, getting good sleep, working on keeping a positive outlook, and cultivating good relationships.

I'll give you the case of my patient. I was administering a PRIME therapy to Kathy and going over this information with her. Kathy is a forty-two-year-old accomplished woman in the music business. She said for her the PRIME was like "the ultimate quick fix." I have to admit she was saying this under the effects of the therapy. I say this because most of my patients describe a soothing and relaxing effect when they are getting the IV therapy push, similar to the kind of high or buzz you get from a glass of wine.

So, she is there, super chill, using her bright mind trained to create marketing campaigns for famous singers. She explained that in her experience and understanding of what the PRIME was doing for her, it was fixing her up right there, fast and easy. But she also recognized two unique characteristics. Quoting her: "First, a 'quick fix' that makes you feel as good as this, doesn't usually have a lasting effect. This therapy makes me, and my mother, feel good and the positive effects surprisingly last for many weeks. Second, 'quick fixes' are not usually good for you long-term and this one seems to be good for your health and longevity, as your work has been showing." This is one of the best analogy I heard so far from one of my patients, about what these therapies potentially may bring to you.

Because the goal is not just to live longer, but to live younger and happier, starting not in your eighties, but now. In order to do that, you need to focus on keeping your cells as healthy and young as possible, adopting strategies that help you to turn back your body clock and improve your BioAge (explained in the next section) starting right *now*.

Your Age for Real: Chronological versus Biological Age

You have probably experienced meeting someone for the first time who appears to be much younger—or older—than they really are. Everyone ages at a different rate. Some people seem to age very rapidly while others experience aging at a much more gradual pace.

This is what differentiates chronological versus biological age, also known today as epigenetic age. Chronological age is the number of years a person has been alive. Biological or epigenetic age refers to how old your cells are, which is reflected in your functional capacity and potential lifespan.

How fast your chronological clock ticks is beyond your control; however, your body and biological or epigenetic clock is vulnerable to your actions and can be positively or negatively influenced by your lifestyle. Of course, genetics also plays an important role in determining your biological age and life expectancy potential. Mounting research indicates epigenetic factors can profoundly impact your biological age and genetically inherited longevity trend.

Diets rich in healthy fats, fruits, and vegetables, intermittent fasting, calorie restriction, regular exercise, high-intensity interval training, moderate alcohol consumption, non-smoking, being socially connected, and having a positive outlook on life have all been linked to lengthened life expectancy. These behaviors have been proven to add decades to your life, but more stunningly, decades of great health and quality of life.

Are you now wondering how old your cells are and how fast you are aging? Have you had your biological age calculated?

During the past several decades, extensive effort has been made to identify reliable aging biomarkers that clearly measure individual BioAge and predict lifespan and healthspan.

This has led me to develop multiple formulas and algorithms to calculate your biological age based on your personal medical profile that takes into consideration factors such as medical history, family history, quality of relationships, degree of stress perception, lifestyle, functional capacity, body composition, and other personal and environmental factors that have been proven to influence your chance of healthy longevity.

You can get your BioAge calculated for free by signing up on https://onogen.com/ and filling out the BioAge questionnaire.

Six different state-of-the art technologies are also currently being evaluated as potential types of biological age predictors: epigenetic clocks, telomere length, transcriptomic predictors, proteomic predictors, metabolomics-based predictors, and composite biomarker predictors. Of all of them, telomere length and DNA methylation epigenetic clock seem to be the most validated and promising. Telomeres seem better able to predict lifespan and healthspan, and DNA methylation initially were just more accurate determining cellular age. However, in the last few years, with the accelerated development of new algorithms and artificial intelligence, the epigenetic clocks have become capable of determining lifespan and healthspan prognosis as well. In my case, I am not looking to know how old my patients are biologically, as a static concept. Instead, I am looking for a more dynamic marker. A marker that can reflect what their chances are to live longer, younger, happier, and sexier. A dynamic marker also implies that it changes over time reflecting choices and behaviors that promote healthy longevity. Without a doubt, the new epigenetic clocks and telomeres' length are the best available markers that meet these characteristics. Also, I find the fact that these markers change as our behavior changes fascinating, as it constantly reminds me how resilient our biology is, allowing my patients to easily understand how powerful our emotions, outlook on life, validated spiritual practice—such as meditation, qigong, and yoga—and mental health impact our genes, our biology and our pace of aging. This has also become one of the most important sources of inspiration for my life's work.

Teloage: Testing Your Biological Age by Testing Your Telomeres

As soon as I understood the diagnostic power of telomeres, I started offering telomere testing to my patients. One of them was Mary. She became the first patient in my practice to demonstrate me the power of nutritional, biomolecular, wellness optimization to determine longevity fate.

Mary had just turned sixty when she started seeing me six years ago. She was in menopause on bioidentical hormone replacement therapy. Mary was a very busy founder and CEO of a major corporation in Florida with hundreds of employees. She originally came to me looking for guidance to optimize her wellness and longevity potential. Mary looked stunning. She was not only strikingly beautiful, but also looked younger than her stated age. I still compare her to the Christie Brinkley phenomenon of "I'm sixty and look like thirty, even in a bikini." However, despite Mary looking great and stating that her energy was through the roof, she was complaining of frequent colds and occasional bronchitis. Recently, these sicknesses started hitting her as often as monthly in the several months prior to seeing me. It seemed to Mary that every time she got on a plane, she got sick.

Her profile was consistent with MTHFR C677T homozygous with multiple deficiencies in her biomolecular profile. The highest deficiencies were in B4, B12, copper, and CoQ10 functional values.

Her biomolecular profile was enlightening. It showed us that although she looked and felt what she thought was the top of her game—except for the frequent colds—she had deficiencies or borderline values in many of the thirty-plus different biomolecular factors that we checked. As I have mentioned previously, the battery of tests I use is mostly based on functional testing, which is completely different from the standard testing that most physicians rely upon. Standard testing looks at static values based on the concentration of each molecule at the specific time of testing in an individual's serum. The technology I choose for my clinical evaluations is based on cellular response monitored "in vitro" in the lab after isolating the immune cells from the patients' blood and exposing them to individual vitamins, antioxidants, minerals, and amino acids. By measuring immune system cellular response to growth factors in thirty-plus different medium or artificially created micro-environments this test likely gives us a better picture of the micronutrient specific requirements of your cells. Because immune cells are very similar in composition and basic functions to most of the cells of our bodies, these results can be extrapolated to the specific requirements of the rest of the cells of our body. Cellular biomolecular requirements are key to understanding the unique gaps existing withing your biomolecular core, which should be really understood as the functional core for your cellular optimal performance and health.

Why? How? First of all, scientific evidence suggests that by analyzing these cells and not the red blood cells as other labs do, we get the best representation of your cellular nutritional status and gaps or deficiencies. Remember that red blood cells have one unique characteristic that makes them different from the rest of your body's cells: they are the main repository of iron that they then use to transport oxygen through your body; so, their composition is unique, and the intracellular micronutrient balance and requirements are too, making red blood cell data not the best extrapolation data for the rest of your body cells requirements. Second, immune cells have a four- to six-month lifespan within which they maintain, increase, or decrease their nutrients' requirements, based on demand-supply-reserve balance. As a result, the way these cells react in the presence or absence of each nutrient may represent not only the intracellular micronutrient requirements itself but a good picture of the individual's biomolecular nutritional reserve—at least for the last six months, which is a more accurate test than the traditional one-time static blood test performed by most commercial labs

Going back to Mary, she was found to have multiple functional deficiencies and a major genetic predisposition to poor methylation. In other words, she did not have enough of the keys or methyl factors essential to maintain her immune system and detoxification pathways. Nor did she have the genetic integrity for her telomeres to work optimally. She had shorter telomeres than expected for her chronological age—her chronological age was sixty, but her telomere age was sixty-six. This meant that although she looked and acted like a younger person due to an elaborate routine composed of facials, Botox, creams, and a physical trainer, she internally was not as young, and her frequent colds were just the warning signal that her body was giving her. After getting these results, Mary also admitted to me that her weight was climbing without a clear explanation, as well as her blood pressure. She had cut calories and tried different modalities, but nothing seemed to be working for her. She also confessed that her ability to cope with stress was somewhat decreased, and things were affecting her a little more. Mary also had to increase the dose of her hormones because she felt that she was getting hot flashes again.

We got her started right away on SAMe by mouth and her own PRIME formula based on her profile. This protocol included IV push therapy sessions that were administered every two to three weeks for six months, and then every four to six weeks for the first year, and every three months in the second year.

I also decided to check estrogen metabolism in her urine because she had symptoms of hormone imbalances. Also, the defect on the MTHFR gene has been linked to difficulty in estrogen elimination, increasing the levels in the body of estrogen metabolic wastes that have been linked to cancer. Sure enough, she had them all.

After a year of the protocol, her telomere profile improved dramatically. Despite her chronological age being sixty-two at the time of the next telomere check, her telomere age was forty, with a total improvement in telomere length of 35 percent. Her telomere length was calculated by measuring the mean of the telomere length in white blood cells, using the most validated technology. Her telomere age was calculated by extrapolating the mean of her telomere length to the general healthy population based on an extensive database from published epidemiological studies. This significant telomere elongation was associated with methylation marker improvement like homocysteine and other micronutrients. Her hormone imbalance

Telomeres, DNA, and Immunity: Turning Back Your Body Clock | 107

BEFORE — 1 YEAR LATER / 35% IMPROVEMENT — **AFTER**

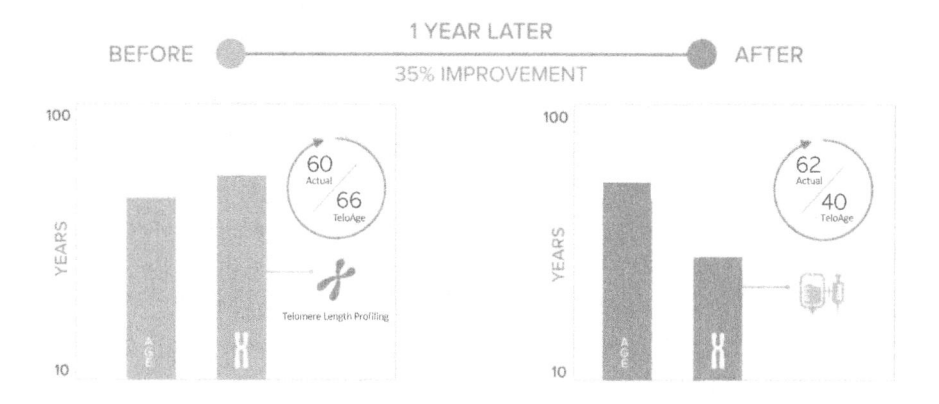

Before: Actual 60, TeloAge 66 (Telomere Length Profiling)
After: Actual 62, TeloAge 40

symptoms faded away while her quality-of-life markers improved, especially in the areas of energy, brain clarity, skin, and hair. She did not originally think she would have room for improvement in those areas at her age, so those were not the goals when she decided to see me. This happened at the same time that her multiple deficiencies in her micronutrient profile were resolved and confirmed by her repeated biomolecular profile.

The rapid grow of the epigenetic clock database has led to the development of new algorithms capable of providing prognosis in terms of longevity, immunity, and pace of aging. I have now incorporated this testing technology into my practice as part of our biomolecular panels. Proudly I share that my patients keep breaking records, with consistent reports of an epigenetic DNA age much younger than their stated age. These results come only to confirm one more time for me the power that simple epigenetic interventions, like diet, exercise, mindful practices, and biomolecular optimization, have on individual's gene expression, impacting aging and healthspan.

As of this writing, telomere testing and epigenetic DNA testing are the most useful biomarkers of aging. However, they are not considered standard for general medical practice, and just a very few physicians understand them well. Still considered to be in an experimental phase, these tests are not covered by insurance. However, there are multiple laboratories that offer these tests, and many health enthusiasts and biohackers are taking the test by themselves, buying in-home kits online.

If you are one of those individuals who has the perfect lifestyle, following habits that have been linked to lifespan extension, such as healthy eating, exercise, a positive outlook on life, and a close circle of friends, with a low perceived stress level, chances are your telomeres are longer than they would be predicted by your chronological age and your DNA methylation is in good shape too. You could still get the test, but most likely the result would be good, and your epigenetic age and telomere age would be either the same or younger than your stated age.

Nonetheless, I have been surprised a few times to find one of my patients, who seemed to be super healthy and following all the right steps, had shorter telomeres than expected, as was the case with Mary.

However, if you are not one of these fortunate individuals enjoying the perfect lifestyle—like most people in this hectic, modern society—then your BioAge could be higher than your stated age. That means your biological clock is ticking faster than it should be and your cells are asking for help. The good news is your biological clock can be reset and the aging process slowed down or even reversed. My recommendation: get tested and start working on your telomeres today.

Are Long Telomeres Always Good for You?

Part of the scientific community is on a quest for a magic pill that would lengthen telomeres with the aim of reversing aging. There is an ongoing debate over whether overly long telomeres can become potentially harmful. The reason for this debate is that most cancer cells have either too short or too long telomeres.

Currently, we know that long telomeres can be inherited from your parents or can be epigenetically induced by healthy habits and lifestyle.

Most of us inherit telomeres in the middle range, but there are rare genetic syndromes associated with long telomeres.

Epidemiological studies have shown that people with these rare genetic syndromes associated with long telomeres seem to enjoy the benefits of a longer lifespan, and a decreased risk of cardiovascular disease, Alzheimer's dementia, and all causes of mortality than other persons with long telomeres. However, these rare cases also have an increased risk of some types of cancer, such as brain tumors, melanoma, and non-smokers' lung cancers, as well as other types. Initially these studies raised concern about long telomeres maybe not being such a good thing and that they might be associated with an increased cancer risk.

However, what we have learned from additional studies is that both short telomeres and dysfunctional long telomeres may be hallmarks of unhealthy aging.

Based on current science, your telomeres shorten with age—and your nutritional and biomolecular core can modify the rate at which this is happening.

It is well-understood that most malignant, pre-cancer, and cancer cells have long telomeres. This increases their chances of undergoing the multiple steps that generate tumors. But this does not mean that long telomeres are bad. In fact, for most of us, having long telomeres is excellent news—most of us do not have the rare condition associated with these dysfunctional long telomeres.

In fact, most of the long telomeres found in the general population are epigenetically induced. That means they are long because of good diet and lifestyle. This kind of telomere elongation, the one called epigenetic, have been broadly associated with increased longevity and decreased risk of cardiovascular disease, Alzheimer's dementia, as well as all types of cancers.

Please remember that micronutrient environment and biomolecular core optimization with personalized IV therapy and oral supplementation are not the only way to optimize your telomeres. In fact, this has been my clinical observation. I also want to remind you that my research is still in early phases and ongoing. However, many recent studies validate my observations, as well as pointing to simple choices in your lifestyle that may also have the same effect. It is simple—the same lifestyle choices known for their good effect for health have been linked to long, healthy telomeres, so, a healthy diet rich in dark green leafy vegetables, dark berries, beans, nuts, lean protein, and good fats rich in omega-3, moderate aerobic endurance exercise as well as high-intensity interval training (HIIT), and meditation and similar stress management strategies. These are still the most important pillars for your telomeres' stability and length and pace of your biological clock.

Another important observation from my clinical practice and data collection is that by optimizing the biomolecular core of my patients, they not only feel better in all these different areas, but these improvements empower them to incorporate healthy habits and make better lifestyle choices while still maintaining their busy lifestyle. As they feel more energetic, positive, happy, and in control of their stress, their well-being and health start climbing their list of priorities.

There are still many questions to be answered in terms of why this elongation happens, how epigenetic factors influence telomere length, and if epigenetic factors can decrease the risk of cancer in genetically inherited long telomeres.

However, what I have seen in my clinical practice is that by optimizing and rebalancing the biomolecular core, telomeres are not only preserved but lengthened by about 35 percent. I have seen multiple cases like Mary's, and even cases more dramatic than hers, like Pat's. Pat's chronological age was fifty-five with a BioAge extrapolated from telomere length of seventy on my initial evaluation. Over one year of biomolecular core optimization therapy, she improved to a BioAge of forty—along with multiple clinical and biomolecular improvements. Meaning, not just that her telomeres lengthened, along with other lab markers, but she felt younger, healthier, and more energetic.

As per my early clinical research and observations, by optimizing micronutrients, and especially methylation status, of an individual with personalized, close, and wise monitoring, we can epigenetically induce telomere elongation and decreased the pace of aging with all the benefits that this involves.

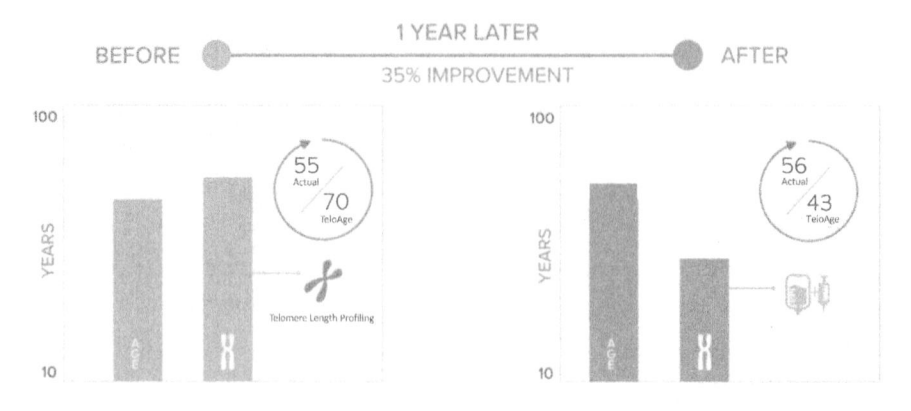

While most biopharma companies are competing against each other to find a magic pill to increase telomerase activity in their quest to find the fountain of youth, we need to be cautious. We know that telomerase, the enzyme that elongates telomeres, has a good side (lengthening telomeres), but it can also have a bad one, like enhancing cancer cell growth and survival.

Remember that lifestyle and interventions like exercise, stress reduction, and nutritional optimization like the ones we have seen with Mary have never been shown to increase cancer risk. Indeed, studies have shown these interventions help to lengthen telomeres and improve lifespan and healthspan, while decreasing the risk for dementia, diabetes, cardiovascular problems, and all types of cancer.

As Dean Ornish beautifully said in his editorial in the *New England Journal of Medicine* a few years ago:

> "Many people tend to think of breakthroughs in medicine as a new drug, laser, or high-tech surgical procedure. They often have a hard time believing that the simple choices that we make in our lifestyle—what we eat, how we respond to stress, whether or not we smoke cigarettes, how much exercise we get, and the quality of our relationships and social support—can be as powerful as drugs and surgery, but they often are. Sometimes, even better."

Inspired by his work and the work of many others, I dare to say that any strategy aiming to optimize an individual's cellular microenvironment and biomolecular core following a personalized approach may become a novel strategy to safely modulate telomere length, improving an individual's chance of having healthy longevity, but also establishing the foundation of the most effective and tailor-made individualized preventive strategy.

Current preventive strategies endorsed by the medical community are really based on diagnostic batteries aimed at finding the most common and life-threatening conditions in their earliest stage, also known as the early-diagnosis approach. Supporters of a more proactive instead of reactive approach, as well as myself and many other experts in the field of personalized functional and biomolecular medicine, are working to shift the current approach to a more sensitive and personalized one that promotes strategies aimed at finding the imbalance that caused the condition in the first place.

This, my friends, should be the real core of preventive-proactive medicine and set the foundation for tomorrow's medicine.

Telomere and Epigenetic DNA Age: Turning Back the Clock

Researchers and clinicians are still debating the best and safest possible strategies to incorporate what we have learned in the field of longevity, telomeres, and DNA methylation into our medical practices. Meanwhile, an increasing amount of data is supporting meditation as an effective strategy to impact and regulate DNA's methylation and telomeres' elongation in a safe, effective, and replicable manner.

This should not be a surprise. Chronic stress, depression, and other negative psychological states can shorten telomeres and change DNA methylation. Meditation has been proven to improve mood and stress management, while impacting gene expression changing the course of different diseases.

Meditation and stress-proofing yourself may change your genes but also your biomolecular profile. The field of mind-body genomics has been making fascinating and promising discoveries that support this and other amazing advancements.

However, there are still many questions to answer, like what do these genetic changes mean clinically? And how do they impact disease prevention and treatment?

While the experts in this field are still deliberating, it seems that meditation and other lifestyle choices conducive to manage stress better, like yoga, tai chi, and qigong, among many others, are safe and potentially positive, which should be enough to empower you to incorporate some of these practices into your life.

Biohacking Your Genes, Telomeres, and Aging

For many years, I devoted my clinical practice and research to innovations in the lifestyle motivational space, but I found my efforts to be futile. I realized that trying to make a modern, successful, and busy human biohack their health by eating right, exercising daily, and meditating consistently sounded easier than it was. Most of my patients were exhausted to begin with and could not find the energy and motivation to even start a healthy lifestyle plan. If I was lucky, I got them excited enough to start, but I could not keep them on the path for long. Life and unexpected situations seemed to sabotage their efforts, and after a few weeks or months, my patients ended back where they had started. They were maybe a little bit better in terms of some new habits, but the reality was that their health changed little to none.

I am not going to lie to you—I had some very successful cases. But I made it my goal to find a solution for most patients, to my Joes and Janes, not to those specific patients who lost many pounds, halted diabetes, and recovered their heart or kidney health. I do have those patients in my practice, but not enough to make me feel I had found the right approach.

It was not until I incorporated the concept of PRIME and RESET that I started seeing results that got me really excited. Remember, PRIME is how an individual covers his or her personalized nutritional and biomolecular needs; RESET is optimizing methylation status and rebalancing inner chemistry and emotions more towards a recovery/healing mode than inflammatory/stress mode.

I witnessed my own patients, as they received their personalized biomolecular therapy, feel younger and enjoy better energy, sleep quality, brain clarity, mood, and sex drive. And when we checked their telomeres a year after therapy, we also saw a significant lengthening of telomeres and improvement of their biological and epigenetic ages.

It is well known that a poor diet, sedentary lifestyle, and persistent daily stress are the perfect formula to speed aging and age-related chronic illness.

Today, most patients know that they must follow healthy habits as they age: exercise, sleep well, eat healthy, don't smoke, etc. But in my experience, it is only when they have their biomolecular core fully replenished that they are capable of managing and coping with stress better; it is only then that they find the time and energy to accommodate all those things—exercise, good sleep, diet—into their lives without feeling they are a burden or an extra task, but instead they view them as a gift.

By understanding the current specific needs of your biomolecular core and by providing these nutrients straight to your bloodstream by intravenous infusion, we may be setting the beginning of a new era in healthcare, where compliance with lifestyle intervention is no longer an unbeatable challenge or an excuse for physicians to skip education and lifestyle modification, going directly to pills.

Medication should always be the second choice in any chronic condition, including pain. I hope that my work can help to reinforce micronutrient therapy as the future of medicine. I considered this my mission. Healing without pills is possible. Moving the standard from "well" to *beyond well* is imperative.

And the best is yet to come. New and better tools are coming along as we gain a better understanding of the power we have over our own gene expression. Tools like peptides. These short fragments of amino acids, normally produced by our body, are key to tissue repair and even gene alterations that occur with aging, stress, and chronic inflammation. Still under investigation, peptides' specific genetic activation powers are one of the most promising therapeutic tools under development today.

While the science continues to develop, there are many tools already available that can be safely incorporated into a personal plan to get you started on your own biohacking protocol. Let's do that!

PART II

THE PROTOCOL

PRIME—RESET—GO

Living a long, healthy, and fulfilling life should be the norm, not the exception. After all, the human body is designed and programmed to heal and repair spontaneously daily. However, we now know that chronic stress and aging progressively compromise our natural healing and regenerative powers at different levels. In order to overcome these challenges I have created, PRIME - RESET - GO, a simple three-step plan based on the latest advancements in science and technology, to help you safely biohack your system and guarantee your natural healing programs are running at their best. Understand that biohacking is combining the best of science and technology to improve your personal health, well-being, and quality of life. These are processes that usually require making small, incremental changes in your lifestyle and adjusting the intervention based on how your body responds to it.

The plan requires that you first **PRIME** your body, by optimizing your biomolecular core. Then you **RESET** your system, switching it from inflammatory/stress mode to recovery/healing mode. Then hit **GO** by biohacking your genes and enhancing specific healing pathways to get them working at their full potential. Your success in this program will depend on how mindful you are through each step and how meticulous you are in observing and adjusting the plan based on your body's response. Improving self-awareness is key for this program. As becoming an active observer of every experience and the effect different foods or interventions may have on your body, energy, mood, and brain power is fundamental for you to learn what works and what does not work for you. I'll be asking you to reconnect your intuition with your biology. The program itself should help you to become a better observer and develop the ability to recognize and enjoy your own improvements, that I have also noticed in my practice is hard for patients these days. We tend to be in the lacking mindset and focus on what is wrong and not what is better, which is not the right mindset if you want to live a long, happy, and fulfilling life. Therefore, celebrating every accomplishment is key as well to keep you right on track for a healthy and happy longevity.

CHAPTER 6

PRIME

Prime is defined as a state or time of greatest strength, vigor, or success in a person's life. It is also the first phase of any painting project, the best piece of anything, and something of first importance. Therefore, I couldn't find a better name for the first step of our plan. The part that will help you to fill in those nutritional and biomolecular gaps that might be compromising your natural recovery and healing powers and expediting your aging processes.

Our goal, yours and mine, is that you find the ideal diet and supplement plan that provides you with all those biomolecular factors you need to fill those gaps and keep your cells up and running at their very best. In the ideal world, diet should be enough. However, due to human spoiling of the soil, food is no longer as rich in micronutrients as it used to be. And to keep up with our demanding lifestyle, many of us as we age may require supplements with extra nutrients, either taking it orally or parenterally—by intramuscular or intravenous shots.

Here are some tips that will help you tune in your diet and lifestyle plan to keep your biomolecular core in tip-top shape.

Finding the Right Diet for YOU

If you're confused about what to eat, you're definitely not alone. Some of the confusion has been driven by changes in scientific knowledge, which has shifted paradigms such as "all fats are bad" to "some fats—like avocados, coconut oil, and eggs—are good." Today, most of the confusion is driven by individuals or groups who parade a certain position, manipulating scientific data to sell you a product. Fads, trends, myths, fake news, and questionable "experts" have become a staple of social media. With the increasing amount of time we spend on social media, it's only natural that our real-world decision-making process is impacted by the friends and influencers we follow. From trying a new recipe or workout we spotted on Facebook to taking a new supplement recommended by an influencer and jumping on the Instagram celery juice bandwagon, we've all let social media impact what we do in real life. I am not saying that regular dudes, models and fitness professionals should not share their advice, but we as consumers need to understand that although these people may want the best for their followers, you and your needs are unique. What may work for them might not work for you and, in fact, might hurt you. The best filter for this has to be you and your own recognition, honoring, and awareness of your unique bio-individuality.

So, next time you feel prompted to try a new trend or supplement that an influencer is recommending, take a moment to question the value of what you learn on social media and whether that influencer has, indeed, too much influence on you without even knowing you.

We are not the only ones who need to evaluate ourselves. Physicians need to as well. We must admit that we share a big part of the responsibility for this phenomenon. We have been so busy trying to keep up with the speed at which pharma and health corporations develop and introduce new products to us that we have left the wellness stage alone for too long. The average physician today is not capable of answering most of the questions our consumers have. Questions on wellness, emotion, spirituality, and sexuality are the kinds of questions that we as the assigned advocates, educators, and advisors of our patients should be willing to answer and help with.

Hey, Doc, what should I eat? My trainer said I should eat small meals five times a day, but I read that fasting is good for longevity. I am confused. What should I do? Paleo, vegan, keto, detox, what the heck is all that? Is it true that sugar feeds cancer? Is it true that eating eggs every day is good for you, even when you eat the yolk? What about organic? Should I have green juices every day?

These are the questions doctors hear daily, and most respond with a vague answer like: just eat a balanced diet, and do not believe everything your trainer says or you read on the Internet. We all deserve better. All these questions need to be answered appropriately, and we physicians need to be eager to learn and embrace this new era where patients are empowered to be part of the decision-making process. Educating ourselves and welcoming every question and input from patients as opportunities to learn more and move on to a more empowering and participative model of medicine. I urge you to choose wisely who you let climb on your own wellness stage. Choose your cast carefully with the responsibility that this important area of your life deserves. Make yourself a main character. After all, without you, there would not be a story to tell.

I am going to try to make it as simple as I can for you. You can have all the questions you have on your mind answered, and you can make eating a pleasurable guilt-free experience again.

Enjoy Your Food

Eating is more than just getting the nutrients you need. Eating is an experience that should be pleasurable and fulfilling. It is an opportunity to break the monotony of your everyday life. It is even an opportunity to make new friends and meet new people, as described by Europeans, a social experience.

Even family dinners have been recognized as being therapeutic to the family dynamic. They are helpful in improving relationships and even kids' school grades and performance. However, for many of my patients, especially those who have been jumping from diet to diet, these social experiences often become a battleground between "tempting" foods and the willpower to avoid them.

Invitations to social dinners and wine tastings are no longer celebrated but seen as a punishment or another challenging test of willpower.

In America, many meals are eaten on the run, and people agonize over their food choices for fear of gaining weight. We all need to understand that as important as diet and ideal weight are for your health, having a satisfying and pleasurable experience every time you eat is health-defining as well.

When it comes to pleasurable eating, the bottom line is to ask yourself first: What do you really want to eat? This is what I tell my patients. It is the only way to create a sustainable, doable and effective personalized plan. If you eat what you really want—not just sometime, but all the time—you will feel satisfied and content faster. You won't need to overeat, because if you want more you can always eat the same tomorrow. After all, you are not starting on a diet tomorrow. You can even enhance the benefits of this experience by creating or going to an inviting and festive environment. Every day? Yes, strive to make eating a special occasion every day. Use your best plate, take your time with each bite, enjoy, be mindful. Use social media for inspiration and creative ideas but be realistic with it. Make your plate beautiful but don't create false expectations, thinking that your plate needs to look like an Instagram post to make eating a pleasurable, fun and festive experience. Remember, it is the festive energy rather than the food that makes the feast. Be festive around food, for yourself and those you love.

Eat Real Food

Benefits of a great nourishing diet are reflected in your cellular and genetic makeup. They help activate natural healing and the immune system. They help your stem cells and other natural regenerative powers that underscore how diet can have an anti-aging and pro-longevity effect.

As expected, micronutrient, protein, amino acid, peptide, and antioxidant demands will be paired up. In order to keep the whole rejuvenation wheel rolling, you need to maximize your intake of macronutrients—especially proteins and healthy fats—and micronutrients—such as vitamins and minerals—and antioxidants during your eating periods.

Your ideal meal plate should be aimed at being half-full with micronutrient- and antioxidant-rich food, which means half full of vegetables. The other half should be left for macronutrients like clean protein, healthy fats, and whole ancient grains. Remember that you are orchestrating all this around whatever you want and like to eat, keeping your promise of nourishing your core while nourishing your soul.

Vegetables

Whole Ancient Grains

Clean Animal/Plant Based Protein

Healthy Fats & Nuts

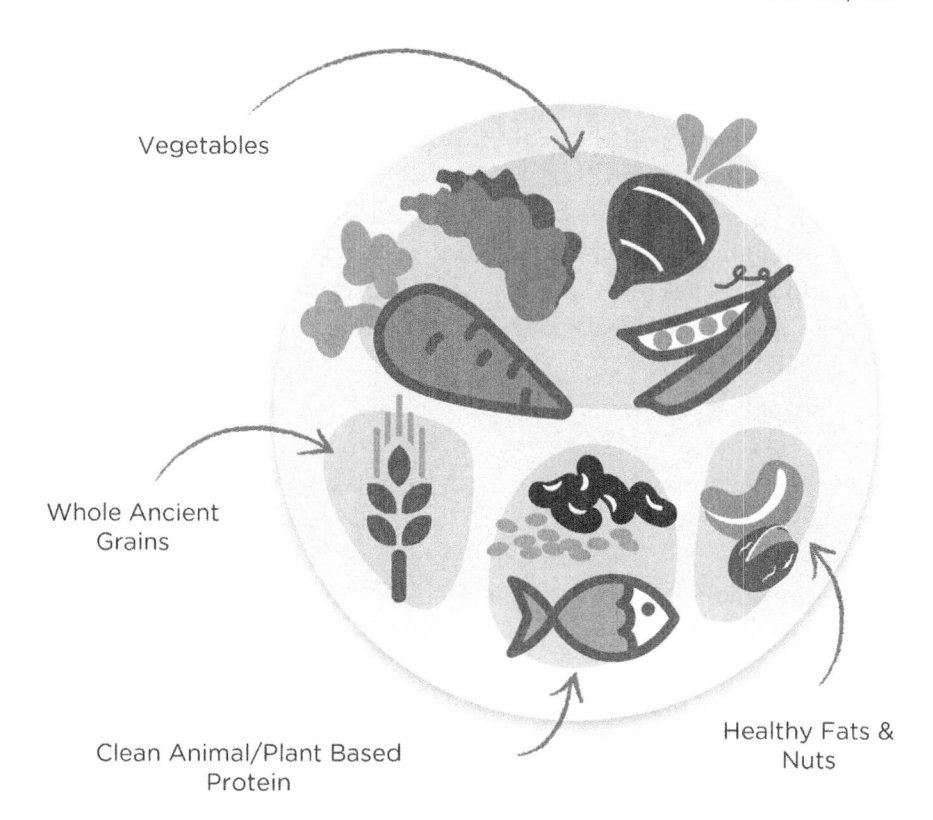

Eat More Fruits and Veggies

Fruits and vegetables are an essential component of your diet. They are naturally nutrient-rich, bringing on more than 100,000 different beneficial micronutrients, such as phytochemicals, bioflavonoids, carotenoids, retinols, isoflavones, genistein, lycopene, polyphenols, sulforaphanes, and so on to your diet. They are also naturally low on pro-inflammatory fats, sugar, and cholesterol.

As most diet programs focus mainly on calorie intake, people tend to count all calories the same and exclude an apple, some blueberries, or even a salad or green smoothie from their diet because they already met their calorie budget for the day or because they bring too much carbs breaking their keto plan—treating then just as any carb or sweet, when in fact these foods work very differently in the body not only in terms of how their calories are processed but also how their phytochemicals impact our body inner chemistry, genes, healing pathways, and metabolism.

For example, blueberries contain phytochemicals called anthocyanins that have been found to improve memory and cellular energy production optimization. Red peppers and tomatoes are rich in lycopene, an antioxidant that may help reduce the risk for coronary artery disease, breast cancer, lung cancer, and prostate cancer. Cruciferous vegetables contain a sulfur-containing phytochemical called glucosinolate, that breaks down into isothiocyanates that have been found to have anti-cancer effects, protecting cells from DNA damage and preventing new blood vessels from growing in tumor cells.

Although even certain phytochemicals are available as dietary supplements, evidence suggests that the potential health benefits of phytochemicals may best be derived from the consumption of whole unprocessed foods. A great example is that while supplementing with beta-carotene was found to increase the risk for lung cancer in smokers, a diet rich in carotene coming from vegetables like carrots, broccoli, oranges, and spinach was found to lower the risk of the same type of cancer in smokers. In their natural state, beta-carotenes are never found isolated but are combined with alpha-carotenes and beta-cryptoxanthin, as well as many other phytochemicals and antioxidants. The surprising finding of this study suggested that by isolating specific nutrients, leaving behind the full spectrum of nutrients chosen by nature and evolution, the beneficial effect might be canceled and sometimes even becoming potentially harmful.

Therefore, because the main sources of micronutrients and antioxidants in our diet are fruits and vegetables, increasing your consumption of fresh and relatively uncooked fruits and vegetables with ten servings a day should be your main goal. However, if you decide to incorporate this beneficial eating discipline into your lifestyle, you do not need and, in fact, should not switch your diet from zero veggies to a whole green diet overnight. In fact, you need to slowly and progressively make the change to help your body get used to new foods and to evaluate which food choices are the ones that work specifically for you.

Although fruits are certainly a great source of micronutrients and antioxidants, some of them are also high in sugar and should be eaten in moderation, using wisdom. Berries are the most beneficial in terms of nutrient-sugar ratio; therefore, they are the group I recommend the most.

For fruits, the time and combination are important, as they seem to be better tolerated and absorbed when eaten combined with vegetables and/or nuts to decrease the sugar spike in your blood which can impact negatively your metabolism and increase sugar cravings soon after. This is one of the reasons why I do not recommend eating fruits first thing in the morning, unless is combined with nuts or in a smoothie with some vegetables. You want to avoid an insulin peak at this time, so your growth hormones, which have been high the whole night helping you to heal and repair, slowly come down instead of crashing down, which is exactly what happens when insulin spike in your blood at this time. We'll talk more about fasting and growth hormone in the GO section of this book. Sugar spikes are also recognized as pro-inflammatory, switching your inner chemistry into survival, inflammatory/stress mode, which we also want to avoid, especially on daily basis, like every morning, so review your morning ritual and avoid making this mistake.

In terms of shakes, I love them, because you can pack many serving of different fruits and vegetables into a delicious, nutritious, and refreshing elixir. I also recommend adding protein to the shakes to improve their nutritional value and metabolic impact. I have even developed some formulas for plant-based protein and collagen peptides that I invite you to try if you are curious. You can find them on our websites: www.onogen.com and www.leafitup.com. Here I share with you two of my favorite smoothie recipes.

The Green

Ingredients (1 serving)
- 6 oz water
- Juice of 1/2 a lime
- 1/2 green apple or 1 slice of pineapple
- 1 cup of kale or spinach
- 1 scoop Leaf it UP Vanilla Plant Protein
- Ice

Directions
1. Place ingredients in a blender, add ice and puree until smooth. It will take at least two minutes. The trick is to put the leaves in first with very little fluid volume and then add fruit to reach a smooth consistency. Drink immediately to take full advantage of all the nutrients.

> **The Berry Blast**
>
> Ingredients (4–6 servings)
> - 1 cup almond milk
> - 1 slice of pineapple
> - 1/2 cup of blueberries (brain fuel)
> - 1 scoop Leaf it Up Chocolate Plant Protein
> - 1 scoop ONOGEN Looking Good Collagen Peptide
> - Ice
>
> *Directions*
> 1. Place ingredients in a blender and puree until smooth. It will take at least two minutes. Enjoy it.

Choosing Your Proteins

Getting enough protein is also important to keep the rejuvenation wheel rolling. Eat enough clean, high-quality, preferably organic proteins, either plant or animal-based, such as beans, quinoa, pea protein, fish, eggs, and poultry.

Note: Choose your fish wisely! Prefer wild-caught small- to medium-size fish, like mahi-mahi, snapper, sea bass, flounder, cod, and haddock, limiting intake of big fish like king mackerel, marlin, swordfish, shark, tilefish, and big tunas. The bigger the fish the higher their levels of contaminants. Note, most canned light tuna is fine, as long as the can is BPA-free and you eat it no more than once a week.

If you wish to get a more extensive list of the kind of fish you may eat, you can check this link from the FDA website: https://www.fda.gov/Food/ResourcesForYou/Consumers/ucm534873.htm

Get Good Fats

Increasing your intake of healthy fats and omega-3s and avoiding saturated fats is also crucial to cellular regeneration and telomere preservation. If you have eliminated completely or cut down severely on your fat intake trying to optimize your health, food rich in monounsaturated fats and omega-3 fatty acids such as cold-water fish (wild-caught Alaskan salmon, sardines, herrings, and anchovies), nuts, avocado, olive oil, and coconut oil should be welcomed back on your plate. As usual, moderation is the key. A handful of nuts, half a small avocado, or two tablespoons of oil is all most of us need.

What about Carbs?

Are you wondering what to do about carbohydrates? First, let me reassure you—it is not just you who is confused about this subject. Most people, no matter what they are doing, are still not sure if they should eat carbohydrates or not. Based on published research and the work of different pioneers in the field of nutrition such as T. Colin Campbell, Dean Ornish, Mark Hyman, Caldwell Esselstyn, and Valter Longo, we now know that carbs are not the enemy. The problem is not the carbs per se, but the carbs that are most available today, as they are very different from the unprocessed, ancient, nutritious grains that our ancestors ate. Our bread is not the same bread that Jesus multiplied, you can be sure of that. That bread was not soft and sweet, but grainy and nutritious. You are better off without any kind of processed carbs. But you can still eat carbs as long as they have been minimally processed and not genetically manipulated. Do you want examples? Cassava, sweet potatoes, plantains, carrots, and beans.

What about corn? First I will remind you that I am from Venezuela, so corn is a staple of my diet. However, I must recognize that most of the corn we find in the market today is not the same corn that my ancestors used to enjoy. When choosing and buying corn, the word organic is just one part of the equation because the way that corn is treated after it is cultivated also determines how good, digestible, and nutritious it will be for you. Corn treated following the wisdom of ancient cultures seems to be the best way to go.

Most corn in the United States is from genetically modified organisms (GMO). Corn is also easily contaminated with aflatoxins, a group of toxins produced by certain fungi that are found on agricultural crops, such as maize (corn), peanuts, cottonseed, and tree nuts, and has been linked to liver damage and cancer. But corn has been a staple of Latin-American food for generations. How did they avoid that? The answer is that their corn was nixtamalized. Nixtamalization is a process by which the corn, as well as other grains, are soaked and cooked in an alkaline solution, usually limewater, washed, and then hulled. This process removes up to 97 to 100 percent of aflatoxins from mycotoxin-contaminated corn.

Historically, society has been using this age-old practice to improve the quality of their raw ingredients, making them more digestible and unlocking certain nutrients for better health. If you think about it, nixtamalization isn't that far from fermentation or sprouting. In many South American regions, nixtamal (corn masa that has been nixtamalized) is still being made in small batches every day. If you love corn and you want to either try a more authentic version of this timeless staple or learn more about these fascinating traditions, I invite you to check out Masienda, a company dedicated to bringing the corn tradition to our tables, at their website www.masienda.com or following their Instagram account. For full disclosure, I have the good fortune to know the founders of this company, and I use their products every time I am in the mood for tacos, tamales, and arepas (traditional corn bread from Venezuela).

In terms of white potatoes, having them occasionally won't hurt you, as long as you don't break your fast with them and follow this wise advice: chill them first. Potatoes have a high sugar load. If you are going to eat a potato, chill it after cooking, then reheat it or eat it cold as a potato salad. Studies show that the glycemic load or index in chilled potatoes is about 25 to 35 percent less than in freshly cooked potatoes that are still warm.

A Few Words About Gluten

Gluten is a combination of two proteins—glutenin and gliadin—found in wheat, rye, barley, and oats. Gluten is present in many types of bread, pasta, and baked products, and hides in processed foods such as beer, hot chips, sauces, processed meats, cereals, crackers, and gravy, to name just a few products.

As more and more people tend to blame gluten for triggering frequent gut disorders, such a bloating and weight gain, there is an increasing number of people avoiding gluten all along.

We know gluten is harmful to some people, especially those with celiac disease, but not everyone who experiences symptoms such as bloating, gas, pain, and irregular bowel habits has a gluten intolerance. They, perhaps, may have intolerance to the way modern gluten is presented to us, but this is totally different.

For a start, the wheat we are eating has been bred, largely at the behest of industrial bakeries and food manufacturers, to have higher levels of stronger gluten. (The more gluten, the fluffier and more voluminous your loaf.) It has also been spread with pesticides and then mixed with multiple food additives and emulsifiers. Products that have been reported as possibly promoting intestinal inflammation by disrupting the barrier between the immune system and the microbiome—the collection of microbes that inhabit our bodies.

So, while gluten need not be a digestive disruptor, per se, it could perhaps become so when encountered in any of its forms at the supermarket, particularly when it is mixed with pesticide residues, food additives, and processing aids that could be troublemakers in their own right.

My recommendation is even if you do not have celiac disease, or any documented allergy to gluten, try to eliminate the processed gluten of your diet anyway and use only products where the grain has been sprouted, comes from organic sources, and has minimal additives. Read the labels, pick the one with the least ingredients and no preservatives.

When buying gluten-free products, follow the same rules of reading the labels and avoiding the products with too many ingredients or additives.

What about pasta? Stick to organic and special occasions and combine it with nutritious vegetables and avoid over-cooking it. You may want to try the available gluten-free alternatives. You might be pleasantly surprised—some of them are delicious.

What About Calories?

In terms of calories, moderation is the rule to follow. In general, for longevity it is advised to reduce total daily caloric intake. Studies on calorie restriction and longevity suggest that by eating around 15 to 18 percent fewer calories than the daily recommended limit, people may increase their chance of living longer and healthier lives. Evidence suggests that such people have better blood cholesterol, glucose levels, and they also have lower signs of cellular oxidative stress.

What About Cleansing and Detox?

Water or juice fasts. Colon cleanses. Salt baths. Infrared sauna. Detoxifying face masks. While many of these detox products and marketing campaigns that claim to rid your body of toxins in a certain amount of time have a very seductive appeal, be aware that not everything out there is good or does what it promises.

First, remember that your body is packed with a sophisticated system to eliminate unwanted substances and toxins. While detox plans and diets don't do anything that your body can't naturally do on its own, using some of these products and strategies wisely can help optimize your body's natural detoxification system.

Second, you are the product of everything that goes through your body. This includes not only the food you eat, but also the water you drink, the air you breathe, and the substances that you put on your skin. You are not only what you eat, but the environment you are in.

Third, you're also a product of your mental and emotional environments. What you see, hear, feel, smell, and taste, together create an impression of the world, and thoughts further refine your perception. If you interpret these experiences negatively, the subsequent chemical and hormonal responses can also act as "toxins" and compromise your health and longevity.

Your ability to understand this concept and put together a plan of action will determine how good you look, act and feel. The plan needs to allow you to decrease your overall exposure to toxins and keep your natural detoxification system running smoothly while still enjoying a balanced and happy life. I have put together some tips that I have learned along the road to keep your system rolling and your microenvironment clean and beneficial.

Eat Clean

"You are what you eat." Unfortunately, I learned this lesson the hard way, but hopefully you can do it differently. Please understand that foods, even the healthy ones, may have more toxins than you think. Although the biggest culprit of toxic exposure is processed foods, be conscious of the presence of pesticides in fruit and vegetables.

Processed foods are full of additives and preservatives, as well as loaded with sugar and sodium. Vegetables and fruits may be coming from contaminated soils and probably have been sprayed several times with pesticides to prevent them from being eaten by insects. If insects would not eat them, why would you?

My advice: read labels, stick to the products made from the fewest ingredients, and avoid processed food as much as you can. Eat more vegetables and fruits but try to stick to the organic section—and please wash your products thoroughly. Organic produce is grown more mindfully, avoiding the use of harmful pesticides and in soil that is more nutritionally rich, but it may still have been contaminated on its way to you, so wash them too.

According to the Environmental Working Group (EWG)'s analysis of test data from the Department of Agriculture for our *2021 Shopper's Guide to Pesticides in Produce*™, nearly 70 percent of the produce sold in the United States comes with pesticide residues. After analyzing the USDA data, the EWG produces two different lists each year, one known as the Dirty Dozen™, which is the annual ranking of fruits and vegetables with the most pesticides, and the other one is known as the Clean Fifteen™, the fruits and vegetables that have few, if any, detected pesticide residues.

EWG'S Dirty Dozen for 2021:

1. Strawberries
2. Spinach
3. Kale
4. Nectarines
5. Apples
6. Grapes
7. Peaches
8. Cherries
9. Pears
10. Tomatoes
11. Celery
12. Potatoes

EWG'S Clean Fifteen for 2021:

1. Avocados
2. Sweet corn
3. Pineapples
4. Frozen sweet peas
5. Onions
6. Papayas

7. Eggplants
8. Asparagus
9. Kiwis
10. Cabbages
11. Cauliflower
12. Cantaloupes
13. Broccoli
14. Mushrooms
15. Honeydew melons

The Shopper's Guide is a resource designed to help you reduce your pesticide exposure as much as possible by indicating which produce to buy organic and listing conventional products low in pesticide residue. You can find more info at ewg.org website.

Most processed foods typically contain one or more ingredients derived from genetically engineered crops, such as corn syrup and corn oil made from predominantly GMO starchy field corn. Yet GMO foods are not often found in the fresh produce section of American supermarkets. According to the USDA, a small percentage of zucchini, yellow squash, and sweet corn is genetically modified. Most Hawaiian papayas are GMO. Genetically engineered apples and potatoes are also starting to enter the U.S. market.

In 2016, Congress passed a mandatory GMO disclosure law. But the final rule released by the Trump Administration, in December 2018, failed to require the clear, simple disclosure of all GMO foods. In addition to exempting highly refined ingredients like sugars and oils, the final rule forced companies to use confusing terms like "bioengineered" and failed to require comparable disclosure options as required by the law for consumers who may not be able to access digital disclosures like QR codes.

These limited disclosures are not required on eligible food product labels until January 2022. EWG advises people who want to avoid GMO crops to purchase organically grown produce, such as sweet corn, papayas, zucchini, and yellow squash.

For processed foods, look for items that are certified organic or bear the Non-GMO Project Verified label.

Be mindful with eggs, meat, and poultry, as well, and try to stick to the organic ones as much as you can. The extra money you invest today will save you money in the long run by preventing undesired health deterioration and expediting healthy aging.

Food packaging is another concern. It is known that plastic containers release chemicals into stored foods and liquids. Two different substances are under scrutiny: bisphenol A (BPA), a chemical commonly used to make plastic clear and tough, and phthalates, used to soften and increase the flexibility of plastic. Both substances have been found to leach minimal amounts of those chemicals from the container into the liquid, entering the bloodstream when you drink or ingest it, especially when the container is exposed to heat. Heating food in plastic seems to increase the amount that's transferred to food. Chemical leaching also may increase when plastic touches fatty, salty, or acidic foods. Under no circumstances should you heat your food in a plastic container. If you need to heat it up and the food is in one of those containers, move it to a glass container or a paper-based container. These substances have been found to be hormone disruptors. So, they may cause hormone imbalances and accelerate aging.

Stay Hydrated

There is no question about water being essential for life and the key to optimizing natural detoxification. Unfortunately, water can also be an important source of contaminants and toxins.

Tap and bottled water are teeming with toxins. Over 140 contaminants in tap water have been found by the Environmental Working Group (EWG). In addition, over the past few years, studies have shown that pharmaceuticals, like prescription and over-the-counter drugs, are being found in tap water. Some of the most common drugs found in water are antibiotics, antidepressants, birth control pills, seizure medication, cancer treatments, painkillers, tranquilizers, and cholesterol-lowering compounds.

Many bottled waters have been shown to be just as bad as tap water, not to mention toxins that leach from the plastic bottles themselves.

Learn more about the quality of your tap water. Invest in a good filter and minimize your water plastic bottle consumption to reduce your exposure to major water toxins.

Detox Your Beauty Routine

Another hidden source of toxins are the cosmetic products we use. Every single day the average woman applies 168 different chemicals to her skin.

In fact, those products you use every day to prevent aging and look younger may actually expedite aging and speed chronic degenerative conditions.

Common daily-use grooming products like toothpaste, lotion, soap, shampoo, and conditioner are also full of toxic chemicals. Parabens, phthalates, parfums, fragrance, and even lead are regularly used as ingredients in these industries, and many products that are banned for use in Europe are currently allowed in the United States.

Many of these substances have been found to interfere with the body's endocrine system, disrupting vital hormone functions. As a consequence, they may produce adverse developmental, reproductive, neurological and immune dysfunction, increase the risk of cancer and accelerate the aging process. Research suggests these undesired hormone disruptors may pose the greatest risk during prenatal and early postnatal development when organ and neural systems are forming.

Studies are still ongoing to determine to what magnitude this kind of exposure may impact different areas of human health, such as aging, fertility, and cancers. Meanwhile, exercise judgment and common sense when choosing the products you put on your skin because anything you put on your skin is absorbed into your body. Besides eating organic, eliminating processed food and plastic containers from your lifestyle, the most empowering thing you can do to decrease and control your exposure to hidden toxins is to use less traditional commercial cosmetic lines and move to products that strive to use clean formulas with minimal preservatives and harsh chemicals. You can find more information on this on the Environmental Working Group (EWG) site, a complete database of ingredients and products classified and certified based on the published evidence of the safety of the ingredients.

Important ingredients to avoid in your beauty and personal care products are: sodium lauryl sulfate, sodium laureth sulfate, triclosan (found in antibacterial products), parabens (methylparaben, ethylparaben, p-propylparaben, isobutylparaben, n-butylparaben and benzylparaben), mineral oil, petroleum, diethanolamine DEA, cocamide DEA, lauramide DEA, alpha and beta hydroxy acids, talc, lanolin, and phthalates.

EWG has also created a certification program, but remember that the products that are not certified by them might still be clean but may not have been checked yet.

One good example of this is my own skin-care line. A few years ago, as I became pickier about my cosmetics, and after looking around for a skin-care line that satisfied all my expectations, I developed my own line of products. All my product ingredients qualified as safe, but I have not yet applied for the certification because my intention has not been to commercialize this line, but to offer a high-quality product option to my own boutique practice and for myself. You can check my line at onogen.com and leafitup.com.

Detox Your Home

Pollution and chemical environmental exposures while you are outside of your home seem too challenging to avoid. However, you can avoid a lot of them inside and around your home. Did you know that indoor air tends to be more polluted than outdoor air—even in the most industrialized cities? And, since people tend to spend 90 percent of their time indoors, detoxing your home is arguably more important now than ever.

Start by eliminating harsh household cleaners containing bleach and ammonia. These toxic chemicals don't stay in the products but are released into our air, dust, hands, food, and drinks.

Avoid secondhand smoking exposure. Keep plants inside your house and choose cleaning products with all-natural ingredients for cleaning, laundry, and dishwashing supplies.

Change your AC filter every three weeks and use UV light devices to minimize moisture and mold from building up in your ventilatory systems. Incorporate old-fashioned traditions like banning shoes in the home, opening your windows when outdoor air quality is good, and washing your hands every time you enter the house and before you eat. While these practices have been around since pre-industrial times, they've fallen to the sidelines amid our fast-paced, modern lives.

Upgrade your home containers. Move away from plastic to stainless steel and glass.

Think of your house as a sanctuary; protect its energy as you protect your own. Use crystals, orchids, gorgeous plants, essential oils, and meaningful art to bring the vibe you want to your sacred space.

Making Detox Part of Your Life

Detox became part of our life as a family more than ten years ago. Not only did I incorporate this for my husband, children, and self, but I convinced my mom, dad, sister, and in-laws. Ten years ago, detox was not a common concept though, so at the beginning I had to convince them that this was not me going crazy after everything from my baby's open-heart surgery to my mom's breast cancer diagnosis and my own burnout. What can I tell you? This is the story of my life. For as long as I can remember, my ideas have always been labeled initially as extreme or "crazy"—as in coloring outside the lines. I've always moved on a spectrum that goes from being ignored or laugh at, to respected and taken seriously. I've been challenged to prove myself constantly like many other adventurous minds out there, who dare to dream out loud. It was up to only recently that people—even myself—started to recognize my gift for questioning the status quo and began to trust my vision and judgment. So, if you are one of those adventurous minds out there, don't give up, you are just probably a visionary in the making. Keep it up!

Let's get back to me and my family ten years ago, when we were just beginning this thing called detox. First of all, Whole Foods Market was just starting, so there were very few cities where you could find this type of grocery shopping. Thankfully, we lived in Danbury, Connecticut at the time, and there were farmers markets on the weekends, not exactly close by but at least they existed. It also helped that we were already on a pretty decent, mostly plant diet, so we just made minimal adjustments and incorporated the organic idea, and the green juices and smoothies into our lifestyle. My sons were four and two years old then. You might think I had a hard time getting them to go along with it, but gratefully that was not the case. They were happy with the new food adventure and enthusiastically drank their green treat with no problem. Maybe because they were already used to having soups and vegetables, this sweeter version was very palatable for them.

The main challenge was to keep up with the farmers market visits and cooking from scratch, with two busy, full-time working parents. There was not a juice bar on every corner like in today's world, and the concept of a farmer market was just starting to become more popular. We traveled forty-five minutes to get to a farmer market on the weekends and became more mindful when choosing restaurants and places to go, but the options were very limited. As we became more mindful, we realized how hard it was to constantly and consistently avoid toxin exposure in your daily life. We also noticed that taking this to an extreme could jeopardize our happiness. Fortunately, we learned earlier to use our common sense. More specifically, my husband would ask us to recheck our actions with this simple but very wise statement: "Hey hon, we are very healthy and clean these days; we are having a lot of good food and good fitness—but no fun." This become an inside joke, if you understand that the name of my blog and company at that time was Food, Fitness, and Fun.

We all learn throughout this experiment that by becoming too strict, you kill newness, spontaneity, and unpredictability. This is where the "no fun" was coming from. Newness, spontaneity, and unpredictability are essential factors for having fun and even staying in love with whatever you are doing. It probably also helped that we met people so obsessed with the toxin concept that their presence could become disruptive and annoying not only to others who were not on the same path but even to ourselves who understood where they were coming from. Another lesson came from our own friends, as we started realizing they felt sometimes uncomfortable eating with us or inviting us to dinner, because first they felt we would judge their choices and they also did not know what to serve us when they want to cook for us. Those became my red flags and daily reminders that I needed to relax and avoid extremes.

So, I decided to create a twenty-one-day program to detoxify two or three times a year with the goal of allowing me and my loved ones to have more flexibility in our day-to-day living. It is kind of like catching up, so if you are exposed a little extra, you can relax and give yourself a break. So that when you get to your good weeks you will have a chance to get rid of those extra toxins.

I'm not saying that we should not be mindful and avoid unnecessary exposures. On the contrary, mindfulness should be your best advisor in your day-to-day life. However, your health preferences should not be limiting, ruling, or preventing healthy and soul-nourishing social activities.

Of course, you are also going to find that as you become more mindful, your taste in friends changes, and you become pickier about who you spend time with. But not going to an amazing party, trying to avoid temptation and unnecessary exposures is not okay. Going out and having fun free of concern and fear, with friends and family, is more than necessary for your health. These activities are as key for your health, longevity, and happiness as keeping your body and cellular microenvironment clean and free of toxins. Do not try to put yourself in a bubble. Take chances, trust that if you are exposed here and there your body's natural detoxifying mechanisms will take care of it, and when you get back to your clean routine, whatever accumulated will be eliminated when you are being extra careful.

In my years of medical coaching, there is something very important I learned: people need a contingency plan. People need to have room within their own discipline to break the routine and misbehave sometimes. Take those little moments to learn how to be easy on yourself and enjoy it with no shame. Of course, being logical, I am not telling you to go out on a "drug, sex, and rock-and-roll" challenge. But allow yourself to be happy with things that you may not usually allow yourself to indulge in during your daily living. And if you associate this with a little bit of sex and rock-and-roll, even better, as long as you do it responsibly and do not put your life or the lives of others in jeopardy. Letting yourself enjoy certain privileges that you do not usually get to enjoy and learning to be easy on yourself sometimes is very, very therapeutic, not only for your mind but for your cellular microenvironment and biomolecular core.

By committing at least twice a year to a twenty-one-day detox, you give your body a break to catch up and cleanse itself. That means avoiding and even removing known sources of toxins, like food containing preservatives and artificial coloring, plastic containers and skin care products. It also means avoiding sugar, caffeine, gluten, processed food, alcohol, and dairy, while providing your body with extra doses of the necessary micronutrients and antioxidants needed to enhance natural detoxing pathways. So, develop your contingency plan. Allow yourself to indulge and have fun outside of your health plan. Practice and balance spontaneity and self-compassion as much as discipline and mindfulness. This, my friends, can be lifesaving.

If you want to learn more about my 21-Day Mind Body Detox-a-Thon program, visit leafitup.com.

What About Food Sensitivities?

Another important factor that I have encountered while trying to build a comprehensive detox plan for my patients is food sensitivities.

Food diversity has decreased 75 percent over the last one hundred years. Modern people following a healthy diet tend to eat mostly the same every week. This lack of diversity and repetitive exposure to the same food can lead to food sensitivities. Therefore, you can become sensitive to healthy food like kale or spinach if you expose yourself to these foods on a daily basis without alternating your foods.

"What is food to one man is bitter poison to others."

—Lucretius

Food sensitivities can be hard to recognize, even though they might be affecting your health and slowing your natural detox mechanism. Symptoms can be subtle and various, like allergies, acne, and other skin conditions, bloating, constipation or irritable bowel syndrome, arthritis, and weight gain. They can go unrecognized for years, causing chronic inflammation and compromising your healthspan and lifespan.

But how do you know? For many people, toxic foods are hard to spot, especially for those who've already cleaned up their diets from gluten and dairy and feel like they are eating healthy.

Science and technology have made it possible for us to learn more about our own specific sensitivities. Our 21-Day Mind-Body Detox-a-Thon program is specifically designed to help you with that as it is an elimination diet with a rotational menu to allow you to discover subtle food intolerance, decrease gut inflammation triggered by these intolerances, and build the perfect diet for you. However, sometimes I see patients who have already eliminated most of the common triggers of sensitivities, yet they still have symptoms of food intolerance.

Companies like Viome and Cell Science Systems (ALCAT) have developed tests that allow us to address these sensitivities. I often use these testing in my practice in combination with our 21-day Mind Body Detox-a-Thon program to help me create a personalized diet and nutritional plan for my patients.

Although it is true that not all symptoms are explained by your diet and what is happening in your gut, the evidence has proven that your gut and the bacteria that live there, known today as the microbiome, are more important for your health than what we ever thought. Gut and microbiome imbalances can manifest way beyond your gut and have an impact on your energy, brain clarity, mood, and immune system. Your food choices are as important or even more important than probiotics. We know that food can alter your microbiome faster than we ever thought.

There are multiple ways to start if you want to optimize your natural detox mechanism. Many people like to focus on the liver, but the gut is definitely as important as the liver in this process. In a society where gut disorders, such as heartburn, bloating, irritable bowel, indigestion, diarrhea, and constipation, have become more prevalent, it is imperative we take care of our gut in order to optimize our detox experience.

Therefore, I have created powdered formulas to enhance the benefits of the 21- Day Mind Body Detox-a-Thon and that address the expected increased demand on micronutrients that are required for the main organs involved in multiple detox pathways, including the gut, liver, skin, and kidneys.

You can decide to take a Viome test, or any of the multiple food intolerance tests available on-line as in-home testing today, or you could go for an elimination and rotational food schedule. Which means, you rotate food, so you don't eat the same food more often than four days apart. And you keep a food journal to take notes of how you feel each day in order to figure out which foods are causing you trouble. Each strategy is good as long as you commit to it and stick with it for at least twenty-one days.

If you need help, you can check on my 21-day Mind Body Detox-a-Thon plan on leafitup.com. I have incorporated all these concepts into a twenty-one-day plan. Make sure you talk to your doctor before you get started to make sure that a twenty-one-day mind-body detox program is right for you or call us and talk to any of our health specialists.

Tweaking Your Diet Just for You

Once you have cleansed the system, you need to ensure that you keep providing your body with the necessary micronutrients to keep it that way. But what is important is that we all need to keep the body clean and healthy. Is it a specific supplement or diet that would help you achieve that? The answer is: we all have a biomolecular individuality, and our needs are as unique as our genes. Therefore, there is no such thing as the perfect diet for everyone or the "one diet fits all."

This means you need to try multiple things until you find the one that works best for *you*. In that process, you need to try different foods and schedules. When adding new food options to your plate, I want you to be aware of how these foods make you feel because one man's food could be another man's poison. So, berries may not be good for everyone. If you feel something disagrees with you, just don't eat it and try something else. This self-awareness is crucial to creating your ultimate personal plan.

Finding the perfect eating discipline for you may take multiple attempts and trial-and-error, until you tune it to the perfect formula for you. This will be the right formula for you at that time, but it will need to grow and evolve with you as your biomolecular core and needs change.

There are genetic studies and food intolerance studies available to help you expedite your ideal diet discovery process. I utilize them, because I have faced challenging cases throughout my career practicing personalized biomolecular and functional medicine. If you want to learn more about this testing, I invited you to check out these websites: www.viome.com, www.pathwaygenomics.com, www.trudiagnostic, and www.alcat.com.

Every step you take toward finding your personal formula moves you one step closer to the ultimate goal of achieving your own *beyond well* status and aging towards a better version of yourself turning back the clock, living younger longer, unlocking your highest potential, and fulfilling your dreams.

But don't forget! In the pursuit of perfection, too much of a good thing is not good anymore. This applies to discipline too! The main rule is to enjoy your meals. Eat what you want and pair it with what you need. Bon appétit!

Using Technology to Find Out What Your Core Is Missing

After all these years trying to optimize my patients' health from their core out, there is one thing I can say without a doubt: everyone's core is missing something. In fact, more often than not, more than just one thing.

Imagine an engine trying to work with missing pieces. Could it work the same? Could it perform optimally?

Unfortunately, when your core is missing pieces, it does not make noises or light up on your dashboard to let you know, but it prevents you from performing at your highest potential. It prevents your mood from being positive and happy. It prolongs your recovery time from work, exercise, and even after illness or surgery. It also compromises your digestion and metabolism, giving you early signs of malfunction like weight gain and postprandial bloating. And what do we do? We blame aging or stress. These missing pieces also jeopardize your capacity to cope with stress, limiting your capacity to overcome challenges, and preventing you from succeeding in whatever you have set your goals for. These missing pieces can speed the aging process and sabotage your natural regeneration, maintenance, and healing mechanisms. A malfunctioning core prevents you from performing at your maximum potential and being as happy as you desire to be.

As if that's not bad enough, if the missing pieces are left alone and the early signs of core malfunction are ignored—as our current medical model does—this malfunction in time causes imbalances: overworking some areas of the core to compensate for the missing parts, creating new increased requirements and more imbalances. In other words, more missing pieces cause a catastrophic ripple effect that eventually manifests as a disease or major health problem, such as hormone imbalances, infertility, asthma, allergies, depression, anxiety, insomnia, colds that progress to pneumonia, herpes reactivations, chronic fatigue, autoimmune disease flares, diabetes, hypertension, heart disease, dementia, and even cancer.

So, how do we know what we are missing to stop this from happening?

Unfortunately, there are not many options. One of the main challenges we have as physicians is that the standard diagnostic tools and testing available today are not designed to look for these subtle flaws.

By looking at your blood with current standard testing, we get different values that reflect the levels of certain molecules in your blood at the time of testing. In terms of nutrients, these values are usually a reflection of what you have eaten the day before but not a reflection of your cellular reserves or functionality. This means that the current standard tests we are supposed to rely on to assess those missing pieces are unreliable and inaccurate. Most physicians are left with primitive, one-time, static vitamin testing to assess the complex function of our biomolecular core, and recommendations are based on the current standard dietary reference intakes, known as DRI.

Current DRI were based on studies performed in the previous century, when people worked eight-hour shifts, took naps, and had lunch at home—a very different lifestyle and biomolecular requirements than the ones for our hustler culture. Their food also came from rich, nourishing, and clean soil, delivered fresh from local sources—many times even picked from the trees in their own backyard. Therefore, their micronutrient requirements were lower while their daily intake was higher, which tells me that the current DRI are obsolete and need to be reviewed.

Trying to fill this gap, biotech companies have brought new testing and have started a genomics era that makes genetic testing openly available to consumers. Today you can spit in a vial, send it out, and get a cool packet that contains the vitamins you need for your specific goals. Although I applaud the initiative and enthusiasm, and I agree with the philosophy of personalizing supplements based on individual genetic characteristics, this is only one part of what needs to be taken into consideration to develop a customized plan for you.

Your genes are a better predictor of your chances of developing certain problems or deficiencies than a real reflection of your current biomolecular, intracellular nutritional status. Looking at only genes when trying to figure out individual nutritional requirements is like reading reviews online about what to pack for your first trip to Mt. Everest. You read and take notes of what most people recommend, but then you must revise the list and create your own based on your unique needs and current climate conditions to get to a better result. Even though you have done that, chances are that when you arrive and start your own journey, you will realize there are other things that you might need. So, you adjust your list again for your next trip based on that. Your list might be helpful to your son, if he decided to go later; however, his list would need adjustment as well based on his unique needs.

This is exactly what I'm talking about. Your requirements are unique based on your individual biomolecular and genetic needs. Using only your genes to determine your personal needs for optimal health is far from optimal, as it's just a prediction of what you might be missing, but not a true current picture of what is happening functionally in your core.

Testing matters, and it matters big-time. Unfortunately, looking at the current values of micronutrients in blood, like when your doctor checks your levels of B12, folic acid, and vitamin D with the standard lab tests, does not give you the right answer either. These studies are designed to look at the current level of the specific vitamin in your blood, which is highly influenced by what you have eaten. It is not even close to what your cell reserve might be and very far from what is really happening in your biomolecular core and cellular microenvironment.

Looking to fill this gap, some scientists discovered that by growing immune cells known as lymphocytes in the presence or absence of different nutrients, they can detect functional intracellular deficiencies of vitamins, minerals, amino acids, and antioxidants. Using these methods may give us a functional picture of the intracellular nutritional reserve, specifically how your cells would work in your body in the presence of more of the specific biomolecular factors. These represent, in my opinion, a vast improvement from the one-time, static number that is the current standard in medicine.

I have incorporated this testing into my practice and use it in combination with serum and intracellular micronutrient and genetic testing to design the IV biomolecular formulas, diet recommendations, and supplement plans I give to my patients.

The test is not perfect. I am sure the technology will evolve from what it is right now. One of the downsides is that it takes at least two weeks for the results to come back, and that in the presence of immune deficiencies, sometimes the lymphocytes may not grow or the number of lymphocytes may not be enough for the study to provide results. However, compared to what is currently available, this technology is the best tool to get the closest picture of what is missing from your biomolecular core available in the United States This technology has been a determinant for the progress of my own work.

You can find more information about micronutrient testing testing at Vibrant America, Spectracell Lab and Cell Science System Lab. (website: www.vibrant-america.com/micronutrient/, www.spectracell.com and https://cellsciencesystems.com/patients/cna/.) Please note the brackets for the websites.

We are currently developing a software platform that will translate these deficiencies into a list of the supplements and strategies you need to get your cellular reserve to optimal levels. You can also bring the results to your doctor or use one of the companies' trained, registered dietitians to interpret the results for you and give you guidance on how to get your core working better for you.

If having blood work does not sound exciting for you, don't let this stop you. You can still get an idea of what you are missing by filling some of the clinical and sensitivity questionnaires available today or even from simpler and more standard blood work. For example, if a test shows that you're anemic and your red blood cells are bigger than they should be or your homocysteine is high and your physician prescribes B12 and folate for you, this is personalization. However, if you decide to take glucosamine because research shows it can be good for joints, you may be stacking the odds in your favor, but this is not personalization. This approach may or may not work for you. This kind of thinking can lead you to buy multiple things, ending up with a lot of different bottles of supplements in your cabinet and taking more than you really need, which is expensive and can potentially cause undesirable biochemical and biomolecular imbalances. The key to making any finding worthwhile is to work with a good physician or healthcare expert, or with a company that can support its recommendations with credible studies and data. As I said before, it is not only biohacking, but biohacking responsibly, that counts.

Get Your Core Fixed and Working at Your Own 100 Percent

Once you have an idea of what you are missing, you need to decide how you are going to fix it. Do you want to take supplements? Which company are you going to choose and which route? By mouth, intravenously, intramuscular, topical? The options are plentiful, and there are benefits and downsides to any approach. You just have to decide which one may work for you best and give it a try.

It is very important to understand that if you are going to get your replenishment just by mouth, the consensus of the experts in this field is that you will need to take the recommended vitamins and supplements on a daily basis for at least six months to one year.

The major challenge I have encountered in my practice when I recommended vitamins and supplements only by mouth is that most patients develop, sooner or later, gastrointestinal intolerance. This is one of the top challenges to patients' adherence or compliance.

It has been calculated that adherence to taking medication—even in people who have been taking medication for many years—is less than 50 percent. Nobody likes taking pills every day; although some do it regularly, most don't. On the other hand, one of the most common side effects of taking any kind of pill is gastrointestinal discomfort. This is also one of the factors that affects adherence and compliance to daily intake.

I also need to remind you that supplements and vitamins aren't a substitute for a healthy diet, so your efforts to eat healthy and nutritious food should be a priority.

However, unless you are eating wild, fresh, whole, organic, local, non-genetically modified food grown in virgin mineral- and nutrient-rich soils and not transported across vast distances and stored for months before being eaten; unless you are working and living outside, breathing only fresh unpolluted air, drinking only pure, clean water, sleeping nine hours a night; unless you are moving your body every day; unless you are free from chronic stressors and exposure to environmental toxins—as described by the Father of Functional Medicine, Dr. Mark Hyman, in the *The UltraMind Solution,* you need to take extra vitamins to meet your requirements to stay at the top of your game.

Our gut has also changed. Vitamin absorption may not be as good as you need it to be to get your core working back at *your* 100 percent. After analyzing and gathering all the scientific facts and evidence available, I have chosen the intravenous (IV) approach as my first choice to treat my patients' deficiencies and compensate for the gap in their cores faster and more effectively.

At least 85 percent of my patients report significant improvement in one or more of the following areas: energy level, mood, brain clarity and/or sex drive, just after the first session. I can assure you after practicing mainstream medicine for twenty years that you do not get this impressive and promising therapeutic response with any other therapeutic approach. This is why I have turned my practice toward these amazing developments and am enthusiastically bringing this approach to more people.

I am not saying these results cannot be accomplished with oral or topical supplementation or even with just diet and lifestyle. I don't doubt that if we were to check His Holiness the Dalai Lama's biomolecular and telomere profiles, the results would be nothing less than stunning. Unfortunately for most of us, having such spiritual wisdom doesn't come naturally. Most of us struggle to keep up with the pace we are living these days. As I'll discuss later, it is more a choice than a duty in most cases. In order to keep this pace without allowing our biomolecular core to wear down, we need a deep understanding of our biomolecular needs and make sure to meet them consistently, either orally, topically, or by periodic IV therapies. The choice is yours.

Meanwhile, I am conducting more research and collecting data to continue contributing to our understanding of micronutrient therapy. I am convinced this is essential to building the foundation of future medicine. While it is easy to recognize that medicine needs to be reshaped, the foundation needs to support a proactive, personalized, patient-centered, compassionate, empathetic, and loving approach.

As part of my commitment to contributing to this process, I have written this book, and I have hooked up with an amazing IT team working on developing an artificial intelligence platform to help us to achieve this vision. I want to thank you for doing your part and spending time reading my ideas. Empowering yourself with new knowledge and sharing with loved ones and even your own doctors is the way we all can contribute to reshape medicine for the better.

"Be the change you want to see in the world."

—Mahatma Gandhi

CHAPTER 7

RESET

Once you have primed your body it is time to reset your system, switching it from survival, inflammatory or stress mode to recovery and healing mode. Always remembering stress is not all negative. It is the fuel that allows us to achieve goals and thrive professionally and personally.

Aggressively and passionately enterprising during the day is great, sometimes sexy, and conducive to success and fulfillment. But, just as with your cell phone, your body needs to recharge, and your software needs to update. Running around nonstop and performing damage control all day long without doing anything to disconnect, decompress, and shift to recovery mode will eventually cause you to burn out, which can compromise not only your professional performance but also your biomolecular core, immune system, and genes. Just as elite athletes need to schedule good-quality recovery time in their routine, so do you. Developing a good, unplugged, and unwired routine is key.

Sleep also gets compromised when you don't develop a good strategy to move from stress to recovery mode. As we have already discussed in-depth in the first part of this book, stress wears out your biomolecular core, creating a vicious cycle where each element intensifies and aggravates the others, leading inexorably to a worsening of the situation.

Today we get easily trapped in the "go-getter or hustle culture." Living by mottos like: "Hustle harder" and "Don't stop when you are tired," you grow so accustomed to being on autopilot that you lose connection with your own biological recovery cycles. We all agree that hard work is good and conducive to great things; however, studies show that unplugging from the mindless race and focusing on the current moment, rather than on what would happen if you don't finish the project, can boost your productivity, creativity, and problem-solving abilities. You know that you solve more problems when you are calm, so cultivate your healing and repair systems.

Don't succumb to internal and external pressure frantically and mindlessly. Please leave the race behind and become the master of your life. Don't be a slave to your daily "to-do" list and external circumstances—I've been there and done that. Don't let irrational emotions take control over your rational thoughts. Gain control of your life and destiny. Move from survival mode to recovery mode. Move from hustler to master!

Make "stay calm" your new motto. Calm brings clarity, confidence, courage, curiosity, creativity, compassion, kindness, connectedness as well as better health, energy, mood, brain clarity, sex drive, and orgasms. The master state fosters mindful productivity and conscious choices in life and work. It also increases your ability to take on challenges with calm and clarity and see them as an opportunity to grow, learn, and develop new skills.

The greatest new leaders are masters not hustlers. By connecting to your needs, you also connect with your natural recovery systems, which is the only way you can responsibly biohack your mind and body. But getting there will take trial and error to develop your own perfect formula.

What seems to be standard for most of us is that anything that enhances your body's production of happy chemical factors, such as endorphins, dopamine, serotonin, and oxytocin, not only make you feel good and happy, but also help your system reset from survival/stress/inflammation/go-getter mode to recovery/healing mode. Cultivate processes that guarantee your system reboots, allowing you to perform at your very best without sacrificing your health and longevity in the process.

Find the Exercise That Makes You Happy

If you ever felt high after a good workout, you know what I am talking about. Endorphins are the neurochemical molecules responsible for this feeling-good effect. Endorphins are produced by the central nervous system and the pituitary gland. Since they act on the opiate receptors in our brains, they reduce pain and boost pleasure, resulting in a feeling of well-being. Endorphins are released in response to pain, but they're also produced during activities like eating, exercise, or sex.

Endorphins are also a natural signal to move from stress mode to recovery mode, enhancing healing and recovery pathways. There is no question that exercising correctly can slow the aging process and enhance natural healing. Evidence already supports physical activity making a significant difference. To prove my point, I invite you to think of those seniors in your life who look amazingly younger than their stated age. Ask them what they are doing. In most cases, their responses are usually one or more of the following lifestyle practices: they watch what they eat; they are active and many times more fit than their peers, and some of them are even impressively ripped, even more than younger friends and acquaintances; but most importantly, they are less likely to have the typical and common aging-associated functional decline and degenerative chronic conditions that affect most of their out-of-shape peers.

What do these fit seniors have most frequently in common? They are active. They are in constant motion!

Rousing numbers of studies have shown that the more active and in motion people are, the less their cells appear to age. These studies have found that active people tend to have longer telomeres than their sedentary counterparts, and when their telomere age is measured, the difference in telomere age is consistently up to nine years. This explains why active people look and feel younger than sedentary and inactive people. The new epigenetic clocks support all these finding as well.

More recent studies show there is a clear dose-response relationship between in-motion behaviors, telomere lengths, and epigenetic DNA age. Although exercise intensity seems to be an important factor—greater vigorous physical activity appears to be the most beneficial and bring the best benefits in telomere length—some evidence also suggests that even as little as moving out of inertia, standing up frequently, and reducing sitting time may also be beneficial for your telomeres.

Cardio Versus Weight Training

The exercise modality seems to matter as much as the intensity when analyzing the evidence of exercise's anti-aging effect. A recent study published in the *European Heart Journal* suggests that exercises such as running, swimming, and biking are better for aging than strength and weight training.

In this study, healthy and previously inactive individuals were assigned to four different groups. One group was assigned to practice endurance training consisting of continuous jogging. The second group was assigned to high-intensity interval training (HIIT) that included a warmup, four bursts of four minutes each: one alternating intense and slow running, walking or resting, with the sequence repeated four times, and a cooldown at the end of the full workout. The third group was assigned to weight or resistance training entailing circuit training on eight machines working to strengthen abs, the back, arms, and legs. Each person in these groups completed three forty-five-minute sessions per week. A fourth group of participants continued to lead an inactive life.

Results showed that on both endurance and high-intensity training groups, people's telomere length increased significantly, which is a sign that by practicing endurance or HIIT three times a week, you may slow your cellular aging and even reverse it. However, weight training did not have the same effect.

Although these findings do not indicate that weight training positively influences your telomeres, this does not mean that weight training does not combat aging or influence your telomeres long-term. This study was measured on previously inactive individuals who exercised for six months. The effect of weight training may need more time to show in your telomeres. Besides, there are not any published studies—at least none that I am aware of after extensive review to write this book—that looked at telomeres, addressing the relationship of lean muscle mass content and telomeres.

This is one of the reasons that research results need to be analyzed carefully and presented responsibly to the public so it is not misinterpreted.

Strength or weight training, like any other workout, has its own benefits, improving fitness and being key to preventing aging-associated muscle and bone loss, another hallmark of aging.

This is just another indication there is no such thing as the perfect study and/or biomarker for anything. Despite that, telomeres and other biomolecular measures are important in evaluating the aging process. It is imperative to understand that the medical profiles that include factors such as fitness and body composition are important for an accurate estimation of your body age.

Laboratory data should never substitute for a thorough clinical evaluation and medical profile—not even in the future with the incorporation of artificial intelligence (AI) into medicine.

It is important to understand, when planning your fitness routine, that differing types of exercise work synergistically. They certainly lead to different but overall benefits that impact our aging in various ways.

Based on current evidence, some kind of resistance training such as weights, plyometrics, or Pilates, should remain a part of your training routine, but they should not be used in place of endurance training. Rather, they should be a complementary form of exercise.

What About Yoga?

Without a doubt, yoga is an increasingly popular form of exercise in the United States. As of this writing, about 4.9 million children and 35.2 million adults are practicing yoga in America.

Yoga, originally an ancient Indian practice, has been established as a straightforward alternative way of exercise involving stretching and holding poses that strengthen muscles. The soaring popularity of yoga studios, activewear, and even a fashion trend, proves that yoga has come to stay.

Yoga as an exercise modality has been extensively studied and has been associated with the generic benefits of any other exercise modality in terms of calorie-burning and cardiovascular health. This includes suggestions that frequent practice can improve the clinical profile of patients with various conditions, such as depression, obesity, hypertension, asthma, type 2 diabetes, and cancer.

The advantage of yoga over other exercise modalities is its relaxation or spiritual component. This "spiritual" twist has been a target for irresponsible marketing using mysticism and false claims to sell yoga as the cure for many ailments with no real evidence.

This is unfortunate, as the benefits of yoga are plenty, and the evidence to support them is on the rise.

From stress relief to flexibility to overall well-being to possible delayed aging, every day we learn more about the real health benefits and the impact of this ancient practice on our biomolecular and genetic makeup.

Therefore, yoga is becoming less alternative and more mainstream in our society. As a result, more people than ever across all age groups are incorporating it in their lifestyle. As we age, muscles and joints weaken, and range of movement deteriorates. Yoga may be one of the most effective alternatives to the hated and avoided but highly necessary muscle stretching. Stretching helps you to maintain your flexibility, increases your range of motion, maintains overall strength, reduces the risk of muscle and joint injury, increases circulation and blood flow, improves your balance, reduces your risk of falling, improves your posture, controls joint and back pain, and it even increases brain clarity. If all this is not enough to convince you to at least take a class and give it a chance, exciting studies suggest the benefits of stretching and/or yoga not only positively impact quality of life but help people to control—in a natural way—common ailments such as back and joint pain due to degenerative osteoarthritis. It also appears to help healthspan and lifespan.

Another positive trend we see is that people practicing yoga are much more likely to get involved in other healthy practices because yoga promotes a sense of belonging and community lacking in other more competitive practices. This sense of community brings two additional well-known benefits conducive to healthy longevity: these communities tend to promote sustainable and healthy living and eating; they also cultivate human qualities such as kindness, tolerance, compassion, and altruism, building supportive and healthy communities and social relationships. Furthermore, being part of a supportive community and having good social relationships has been linked to health and longevity, demonstrated by epidemiological and centenarian studies—studies conducted in populations where people live up to one hundred years!—but also by studies that found longer telomeres in those fortunate people who have cultivated friends and relationships that make them feel supported.

In spite of the positive effects of yoga and stretching on longevity and multiple aging-associated diseases broadly demonstrated in several studies, a clear understanding of the mechanism of these benefits is still being investigated. However, there is evolving evidence that regular practice of yoga and meditation stabilizes telomeres, increases oxygen flow to the cells and reduces stress levels by modulating the brain-adrenal axis or hypothalamic–pituitary–adrenal axis (HPA axis).

There is also accumulating data that practices such as yoga and meditation can help to maintain not only telomeres, but also DNA integrity in general. Several studies, including one from Harvard Medical School, have suggested that practices that induce the "relaxation response," like yoga and meditation, can be of key importance to human health and lifestyle disorders.

The study looked at people who had either irritable bowel syndrome (IBS) or inflammatory bowel disease (IBD), including Crohn's and ulcerative colitis. Researchers found that those who performed yoga and meditation regularly for two months had fewer symptoms associated with the two gut disorders. What was more striking was that blood samples from both groups revealed a clearly different genetic makeup among the responders. That is, different genes were either switched *on* or switched *off* in ways that were different from the non-responders. This genetic modulation may help us better understand how practices such as yoga and meditation help reduce stress that is otherwise associated with autoimmune disease flares and reactivation.

In another study published in *Oxidative Medicine and Cellular Longevity*, researchers found that twelve weeks of yoga slowed cellular aging. The program consisted of ninety minutes of yoga that included physical postures, breathing, and meditation for five days a week over twelve weeks. Researchers measured biomarkers of cellular aging and stress before and after the twelve-week yoga program and found that yoga slowed down markers of cellular aging and lowered measures of inflammation in the body.

It is interesting that asanas in yoga are thought by ancient culture to reduce buildup of toxins in the body. It has been hypothesized that yoga may reduce the deleterious and aging effects of reactive oxygen species (ROS) and consequent damage from oxidative stress. Although these hypotheses are not based on scientific data, but rather empiric or intuition, current studies suggest that the ancients were far from being wrong.

Building Your Own *Aging Beyond Well* Fitness Plan

Enough of all the science talk. Let's jump into building your telomere repair anti-aging fitness plan.

First of all, if you are already practicing any kind of fitness modality, you should focus on trying to make your routine more comprehensive by incorporating the three different components most associated with health and longevity benefits.

1. Endurance: in the form of jogging, swimming, riding a bike, spinning, or HIIT.
2. Resistance: weights, plyometrics, Pilates.
3. Stretching before and after your exercise routine and yoga. Most people do not perform enough stretching exercises. Please do not underestimate its importance, leaving it as an optional activity for when you finish your routine earlier or have extra time after your training. Stretching is as important as any other part of your fitness routine, if not more.

If you are one of those who hates exercise, or you have had a negative experience in gyms or in physical education in school, I invite you to give yourself another chance. Start by recruiting a good physical trainer twice a week and move from there. I encourage you to start gently. You can also start by walking around the room for two minutes, building up to five minutes. Lift your arms over your head. Bend over toward your legs, then lift your body upward again. I just want you to retrain your body to move again.

Newton's first law of motion describes inertia. According to this law, a body at rest tends to stay at rest, and a body in motion tends to stay in motion, unless acted on by a net external force.

When you start to move more and come out from inertia, you realize that movement itself is good and you will reprogram your brain, muscles, and joints to what movement is. No matter how you decide to start, start gently, get help and support from people who know what they are doing, and challenge yourself to do a little more each week.

Because people often ask me what I do, I am going to guess you are also curious.

I am a runner, so I run forty-five minutes three times a week. I alternate HIIT with occasional sprints or plyometric exercises like plank holding, burpees, lunges, push-ups, and dip squats. I run outdoors with my dog, Boone, because that is how I enjoy it the most. I also sometimes run with my husband on the weekends. I have run with my kids, but it seems they like other sports better, so I respect that because not every modality is for everyone. The trick is to find yours and keep spicing it up with new things or scenarios.

For example: everywhere I go, every city I visit for either work, or pleasure, I run outdoors while there. It helps me to see more things and breathe in the vibe of where I am. It's just me; I like to run. I am passionate about it. It make me feel free, kind like Forrest Gump when starting running and did not stop until suddenly he decided. It brings me to my peaceful place. I invite you to explore and find your own sport, your own passion.

If you seem to have a hard time finding it, keep looking. If you visit a yoga class and don't like it, ask people there what other places they have been. Dedicate time to this endeavor as if your life depends on it because it does. No matter what, get up from your chair and walk around to stay in motion.

Good luck! Namaste!

Free Your Mind

Stress is expensive. It causes micronutrient depletion, slowing down detoxification pathways while increasing detoxification pathway use. This increases the amount of waste produced by the body. These factors together compromise our natural detoxification mechanism and increase oxidation, speeding aging and increasing unwanted aging-related degenerative processes.

During stress peaks, there is a necessary increase in the production of hormones, such as cortisol, and neurotransmitters like glutamate. For the body to sustain this production, there has to be an increase in micronutrient intake, which usually does not occur. Resources have to be taken from our micronutrient reserve, which compromises the availability of key nutrients and factors for the detoxification mechanism to work at 100 percent. Also, the increase of hormone production and cellular waste associated with stress itself increases the utilization of the natural detoxification pathways, compromising optimal function of this essential mechanism. This can shift the system to an unsustainable backup status, accumulating toxins in different tissues that will eventually disrupt your health and quality of life at multiple levels.

Good health isn't just about the physical body. Our mind and body are interconnected, and stress induced by built-up tension can affect the body and mind tremendously, so detox requires us to address both systems. Just like the body, the mind and soul need occasional, mindful cleansing. It is our job to recognize when it is necessary and open space in our schedules to make it happen.

Emotional toxicity can build in many areas of life—from self-esteem, self-image, sleep, and relationships. If you are wondering why I have included relationships here, research supports the idea that "...we, humans are simultaneously biological and cultural beings." This means we are all interconnected and need to cleanse not only the mind, inner-self, and our bodies, but also our social networks and relationships, including family, marriages, and friendships.

Start with baby steps. Recognize the need to spend more time disconnected from your phone, electronics, and other people. What has worked for me and my patients is to schedule time for oneself every week, time I call "ME time." This means that you disconnect, especially from your mobile phone, and dedicate some time to detox your mind. I usually do it after my running session three times a week. But if I recognize there is extra toxicity building up, I give myself extra time. I have found that it becomes easier for me to shut down my mind and reset my emotions after running, likely explained by the endorphins that are running through my body at that time.

I also like to meditate, daydream, and reflect. Sometimes I just practice passive contemplation. Sometimes my monkey mind cannot stay quiet, so

I just breathe and try to observe it. Every day it changes, as my mind is in different modes. I used to feel frustrated at the beginning of my meditation practice because I thought that I was not doing it right. With time you'll realize there is no perfect way to meditate, just your way. And your way changes every day because your mind is changing. Just like the ocean is sometimes choppy and sometimes calm.

Learn to enjoy and accept every mode of your mind and make your best effort to become an observer without trying to control it. You'll eventually recognize a pattern and learn that the mind, like the ocean, needs to go through different modes to clean itself and keep evolving. Although the days you achieve peace of mind are enchanting and you wish to stay there forever, understand it is not possible and learn to enjoy them when they come. This acceptance itself will bring you emotional healing and the wisdom to continue growing, but it takes time and work. Please remember that the benefits will be worthwhile. As you achieve more constant peace of mind and worry less, your physical health and biomolecular harmony will benefit as well, which will positively impact every aspect of your life—performance, energy, mood, brain clarity and sex drive, relationships, and work achievements.

How Do You Know if You Are in Need of a Mind and Inner-self Detox?

These are signs your mind and inner-self need a detox:

- If you can't stay away from your phone for more than a few minutes.
- If you find you're miserable, scrolling through any social media for hours every day or complaining about your life when talking with friends.
- If you are using sarcasm and cynicism more often than you used to.
- If you feel your heart hurts. Or even worse, if you feel nothing hurts anymore.
- If you can't sleep well.

- If you find yourself shying away from any positive, spiritual, or inspirational activity.
- If happy and positive people piss you off.
- If you can't remember the last time you went to the beach, played with kids, watched the sunset or sunrise, walked barefoot in the grass or sand, or felt the summer breeze on your face.

If you see yourself in any of these scenarios, you are in huge need of a mind and inner self detox. You should not do it alone. I implore you to take a break or sign up for a retreat. The results are worth the work.

Please remember, in your quest for peace of mind, do not make the same mistake I made at the beginning, one I still find myself sometimes making. Do not try too hard! Do not go with the expectation that you are going to obtain peace of mind comparable to the Dalai Lama in the first few years of your practice. You will not. Leave expectations aside and recognize them whenever they are blurring your vision. Use compassion with yourself if you find yourself following what you perceive at the time is the wrong path. Remember, there is no wrong or right path. It is just your own path, and everyone's path is simply different. Just might need to feel "off" a few times to find your own way. Do not give up. Above all, be kind to yourself. Keep in mind that you are always doing the best you can, even when you screw up.

Let go of the ambition to be that perfect being you think you should be. This idea is utterly unrealistic and can put you in a constant state of not feeling good enough, which can affect your self-confidence and your inner self-cleansing process. Most of the junk that creates toxicity in your life is not always avoidable. Remember that your job is not to control what is coming but to work on how you perceive it and manage and learn to recognize when the junk is affecting your emotions and judgment. You must recognize when this happens that it is time to detox. So, take extra "ME time" without feeling guilty or ashamed. The fact that other people do not do it or feel they need it only means they are unaware of the benefits it brings. Give it a chance, and you won't look back.

Here I share some practices and activities that I have either incorporated along my path or learn from some of my patients who have found them useful, so you can try them yourself, with the goal of developing your specific and individual formula to achieve peace of mind while thriving into a healthier and happier version of yourself. But, for these to be truly effective, you need to make this a priority on your daily to-do list. This needs to become as routine for you as taking a shower or brushing your teeth. So, no matter how busy you are you always find time periodically to dedicate to these activities. Get on it as if your life depends on it, because it does. Finding the right formula for you will promote mind and inner-self cleansing while enhancing your life experience and joy and increasing your chance to enjoy healthy longevity, which means living younger, longer.

1. Surround yourself with people who make you laugh and genuinely care for you.

People who make you happy are real treasures. In this modern era, we all struggle between career and family, and suddenly our pets, plants, TV, and bed become our closest and most frequently seen friends. Friendship is an essential ingredient for optimal health. People with a dependable network of friends and relatives are in a better position to deal with stress, have better health, and live longer, as shown in multiple studies. Friends also represent a determinant factor in treatment and recovery of cancer. Research published in *Lancet* a few years ago, showed women with breast cancer who took part in social activities suffered much less pain and went on to live twice as long as those with less social interactions. A decade-long study conducted by the Center for Aging Studies at Flinders University, Australia, revealed that elderly who have a large network of friends tend to live longer by about 22 percent than those who have fewer friends. Cultivate your friendships and treat your friends as your most precious assets because they really are. Find time to celebrate your friendships and enjoy good company, share with them, but do not become dependent on them as this can transform something beneficial to something negative. Our friends, or those we call our tribe, are usually our mirrors. What we recognize and like or even dislike from them, already exists within us. Understanding this on a deeply spiritual level, allows us to ensure the longevity of our relationship with them. We then find forgiving them easy; we understand them better; and we support them unconditionally.

Avoid using friends to fulfill your inner emotional needs—this must come from you. In any relationship, if someone is expecting to get his/her/their emotional needs fulfilled by the other person instead of themselves, the weight of this request becomes eventually unbearable, and the relationship will become toxic and in need of a make-over or termination.

So, laugh, be silly, and make sure that friends and fun become part of your daily routine. Nourish each other and keep it balanced. Recharge yourself in many ways, not only in this way. This will prevent you from falling into false patterns and contaminating your relationships. They are a treasure, take care of them.

2. Smile and be kind to yourself and others.

Happiness and kindness are highly contagious and gratifying. From studies run to determine the connection between emotions and brain function, we have learned that when you smile, make someone feel welcome, witness, or receive an act of kindness, and practice forgiveness and compassion, your brain areas for reward and pleasure light up on brain scans. This specific brain activation explains the rewarding feeling we all get when we help or make someone happy, also known as the "helper high."

On a biomolecular level, the hit of endorphins that is followed by a subsequent release of dopamine and oxytocin explains the "helper high" effect that these activities induce. This effect is not only highly pleasurable but also helps to slowly train and rewire your brain over the long-term to stay in a more positive and happy mode. This mode helps you cope with daily stress and improves your performance in all areas of life. This kind of brain activation profoundly impacts the health of your genes and the length of your telomeres.

It also promotes improvement of an area of the brain known as the hippocampus, which is associated with relaxation and long-term memory.

Every time you are kind towards others or yourself or even smile, you activate important pathways that bring more joy and happiness to your life and the life of others. But these little events are also imprinted on your genetic and biomolecular blueprint, enhancing your immune function and natural regenerative and healing powers.

3. Sleep tight.

Sleep is not a luxury. Sleep is an indispensable essential requirement for our health and well-being. We actually put our health in jeopardy by sleeping less than we need. Ensuring adequate and quality sleep each night is a must to support your body's health, immunity, and natural detoxification system. Sleeping allows your brain to reorganize and recharge itself, as well as your body to remove toxic waste byproducts that have accumulated throughout the day, and sleep allows the immune system to do its regular surveillance and tissue repair. Regular sleep deprivation is also an underlying issue that can promote a multitude of ailments including irregular heartbeat, heart disease, heart attack, heart failure, hypertension high blood pressure, stroke, type 2 diabetes, obesity. Sleep deprivation also increases cortisol levels, makes you gain weight, impairs your judgment and stress-coping skills, increases your risk of feeling blue or anxious, and affects your memory.

Lack of sleep can create a vicious cycle that increases stress; the more stressed you are, the less sleep you get. Getting even one night of poor sleep can throw our hormones out of whack besides the increase in cortisol as stress is increased. Insulin (the hormone that regulates our blood sugar) and ghrelin (a hormone that makes us hungry) levels also increase, explaining why sleep deprivation is thought to be one of the major culprits of obesity.

As stress increases with sleep deprivation, the biomolecular core requirements increase as well, affecting how well you feel and also slowing your natural detoxification pathways, debilitating your immune system, and even compromising your telomere length. Not surprisingly, people who get roughly seven or more hours of sleep a night tend to have longer telomeres, especially among the elderly. People who get five hours or less have much shorter telomeres.

There are other aspects of disrupted sleep that are also associated with shorter telomeres. Sleep apnea creates oxidative stress, a chemical known to shorten telomeres. If you have sleep apnea or snore, and you have not been checked by your doctor or had a sleep study, please do so. Sleep apnea has been linked to shorter telomeres as well as increased risk of obesity and cardiovascular disease.

Sleep and immunity are also tightly linked. Immune system activation alters sleep, and sleep affects your body's defense system, specifically affecting what we know as cellular immunity, which is in charge of fighting viruses and cancer. Who does not feel sleepier when fighting a cold? Nothing like a restorative nap and a good night's sleep to get you feeling better, right? Enhancement of sleep during infection is a natural response of the body to increase your immune defenses. Indeed, sleep affects various immune parameters. Good sleep quality has been associated with a reduced risk of infection and improved infection outcome and vaccination responses.

However, in the absence of an infection, sleep regulates inflammation and tissue repair and recovery. As we have discussed, these key processes are regulated by a delicate signaling system that rules our inner chemistry through the exosomes. Sleep is essential to restore and recover from the harsh effect of your everyday life. Your immune system needs a full night's sleep to complete the surveillance required to keep your body in optimal health, decreasing the risk of developing low chronic inflammation and immune dysfunctions associated with increased stress and aging.

Not surprisingly, chronic sleep deprivation is associated with low-level chronic inflammation, accelerated aging, immunosenscence (immune system decline associated with aging), increased risk of cancer, greater susceptibility to infection, and decreased protection after vaccines. Sleep is also key to keeping your immune memory cells, required for long-lasting immunity, functioning at their best. Furthermore, the circadian rhythmicity of gene expression related to immune function and stress response is also disrupted after sleep deprivation, which has been found to impact negatively your immune system response to viral infection and the durability of your immune memory after infection or vaccination.

Because sleep quality has been shown to be so vital for healthy longevity and strong immunity, just by improving the quality of your sleep, you can be resetting your body to live longer and better., Here are some tips that might help you to create the sleep quality you, your biology, your genes, and your telomeres deserve. Start with one, and slowly incorporate those that sound appealing to you.

Be patient and consistent. If you do not see results, please seek advice from your physician. Sleep is one of the most important activities for your health. Make sure you are getting enough hours and good quality sleep.

- Establish a regular bedtime routine and wake-up rhythm (a must for everyone).
- Eat and drink fluids early, at least three hours before bedtime.
- Limit caffeine consumption.

- Create a soothing transition routine to prepare for going to sleep.
- Unplug from your cell phone, computer, TV, and all electronics at least an hour before going to bed.
- Unwind with mindfulness meditation before going to sleep.
- Engage in gentle and restorative activities like reading, instrumental music, or yoga.
- Try using lavender essential oil to calm you down.
- If you like to read, read a print book instead of a book on a screen. The blue screen suppresses melatonin (the hormone that regulates sleep-wake rhythm).

4. Get in touch with nature.

Research reveals that stress may increase or decrease in association with the environment that surrounds you, which in turn may impact positively or negatively your biomolecular core. What you are seeing, hearing, perceiving, and experiencing at any moment is changing not only your mood, but also your microenvironment and your cellular health and function. This eventually will impact your nervous, endocrine, gastrointestinal, and immune system.

Being in nature, or even viewing scenes of nature, can reduce stress, anger, and fear. Exposure to nature not only makes you feel better but switches your brain into recovery/happy mode, increasing the release of neurotransmitters, hormones, and peptides related to joy and happiness, similar to meditation. This mode contributes to your physical well-being, reducing blood pressure, heart rate, muscle tension, and decreasing or blunting the production of stress hormones.

Research conducted in hospitals, offices, and schools has found that even a simple plant in a room can have a significant impact on stress and anxiety. There are a growing number of studies and campaigns putting forward evidence that a connection with nature makes us healthier and happier people, something that few of us nature lovers would argue with.

A recent evaluation of the UK's first month-long nature challenge, *30 Days Wild,* which involves people "doing something wild" every day for thirty consecutive days, shows scientifically and statistically how significant it really is.

The study showed that there was a scientifically significant increase in people's health, happiness, connection to nature, and active nature behaviors, such as feeding the birds and planting flowers for bees—not just throughout the challenge but sustained for months after the challenge had been completed.

I am convinced that this effect can also be replicated by cooking, manipulating, or eating fresh vegetables and fruits. Don't you feel it? There is something in nature that also replicates in fresh fruit and vegetables that soothes and heals, which explains why in spring everyone is dying to go out, smell the grass, and drink some fresh juice.

> "But man is part of nature, and his war against nature is inevitably a war against himself."
>
> **—Rachel Carson, author of *Silent Spring***

5. Live in gratitude.

> "We often take for granted the very things that most deserve our gratitude."
>
> **—Cynthia Ozick, author of *Antiquities***

How often do you pause to appreciate what you have in life?

Happiness and gratitude are two of the most crucial factors in life. People who live longer and more fulfilling lives are not people who have perfect lives, but who have focused on the positive, bounced back from setbacks, and cultivated happiness and gratitude as one of the most precious elements of their lives.

Happiness is sometimes viewed as a state that can be reached by achieving some goal or acquiring possessions (e.g., "I would be happy if _____."). However, from psychological research we know that happiness is more related to being grateful for what we already have.

Awesome things are happening to us, all the time, every day, even between all the bad and stressful things that happen. Think about it. Just the fact that you woke up this morning should give you enough reason to celebrate. Do you know that your own expectations can eclipse your joy? I always say that one of my masters in gratitude is my own dog. He wakes up, and as long as he is healthy, he is happy. He smells the grass of my backyard every day with the same enthusiasm he had when he smelled it the first day. He runs to his food and enjoys his water. He enjoys the sun, and he enjoys the love we give him. He wiggles his tail every time he meets someone, no matter if he has seen the person many times or just for the first time. What about us? Can we humans develop the capacity to be grateful for those little things? Can we knock down expectations, and be grateful for what we have, while we still keep working to achieve higher goals? Can we be grateful even when those events we may perceive as negative, such as obstacles or bumps on the road, challenge us? After all, aren't those events the ones that have taught us the best lessons? Obstacles and challenges are annoying and many times painful, but they help us to grow and thrive, bringing ourselves closer to the truest and highest expression of ourselves.

I know it sounds weird. It took me a while to understand this. But I can assure you that by shifting your mindset to being more grateful, even for your day-to-day activities, it will make your life happier and more fulfilling. Remember: it is all perception. You can see the challenge as an obstacle or as an opportunity. This changes it all. As you practice, you get better, and as you get better, you become capable of experiencing joy even through difficult circumstances. Start training yourself by looking for the gift in the moment and focusing on the opportunities this obstacle is bringing.

Like anything worth practicing, it can be difficult at first. Over time, it becomes simpler and easier, but to get there you need to commit to the idea of rewiring your brain and creating new circuitry that supports this kind of behavior. This requires awareness and constant attention to your inner state. You will feel uncomfortable at first, but you need to get used to feeling uncomfortable in order to make the changes to really imprint in your brain.

We are all on the road to find our purpose in life and to make our dreams come true. The road is full of beautiful moments alternating with bumpy periods and challenging situations. It is easy to ruminate on the things that didn't go well during the bumpy periods. We lack practice in remembering and savoring the beautiful moments we encounter along the journey.

I invite you to take on a challenge this week. Every day of this week, find a different thing to be grateful for, write it down, and share it with others. You can use email, Facebook, Instagram, or Twitter. You can also take a photo of something, somewhere, or somebody who makes your day joyful and bright, save it and look at it multiple times while recreating the feelings you had at that moment using your imagination, or post it on social media and write about it. Do not wait. Start collecting your joyful moments or serendipities early in the day. You may be surprised that you end up with more than one awesome moment. With practice, you will get better at recognizing these good things throughout your day.

If you would like to take this activity one step further, start practicing shifting setbacks or challenges from negative things into positive things and be grateful for the opportunity and the lesson.

> "Do not spoil what you have by desiring what you have not; remember that what you now have was once among the things you only hoped for."
>
> —Epicurus

6. Get to know your ego.

Ego is your sense of personal identity, your conscious thinking, responsible for your self-esteem and self-confidence. We all interact with our ego every single day. Do not ignore it. Instead, get to know your ego better. Learn what triggers it and what soothes it. Use it when you need it, but do not let it go wild. A wild ego can be very toxic for you and for your relationship with yourself and others.

> "The ego only thrives in the shadow of our unconsciousness. As more of our inner world comes to light under the glare of consciousness, the more the ego fades. So, the path to releasing the ego is to know our true self."
>
> —**Dr. Shefali from *A Radical Awakening***

Your ego is a tool, like a piece of software, allowing you to interact with the world. It is how you make decisions, set personal boundaries, and maintain self-esteem. It is important to prioritize taking care of yourself and feeling good about who you are, allowing you to stand by your values. These are all signs of a healthy ego.

It is when your ego takes over that the wars begin. A big ego makes for a big fool (even if you're not aware of it). Recognize when it is taking over and calm it down. Monologues, inflexibility, and fighting to prove you are right about matters that are not life-changing for you or your loved ones are red flags of a wild ego. Being the one who always talks, not recognizing and thanking the help of others in achieving your accomplishments, not listening, not caring about others but only about yourself all the time, and complaining about your life constantly are consistent signs that your ego needs a tune-up.

Practice taking two or three deep breaths before jumping into a fight or a conversation. Ask yourself if you are really listening and if what you have to say will bring something important to the conversation and to the listeners, or it is just your ego that impulsively wants you to jump in. Put yourself in the shoes of the other person, revise what his or her needs and interests are, and if what you are going to add is helpful to those who are there. Moreover, before you react emotionally to any event or comment involving somebody else, recognize individual uniqueness and understand that everyone thinks differently. Embrace diversity, not only of race, religions, and gender but of thinking and emotions. Be gentle and kind. Breathe, listen, connect with the people who are there, think, and then act. Ego usually does not let us mindfully act but instead wildly reacts. Do not let it do that. It will take time and practice to develop the muscle, but it is worthwhile.

It's important to remember that you are more than just this physical body, that you hold an expansive consciousness within yourself.

And remember, if you feel your boundaries or principles are being violated, and after taking a few breaths you really believe you need to speak up, do it. Just make sure you do not jump straight out of your emotions. And if you do, recognize that you are human. An ego is part of all of us. Back off and get back on track without shaming or beating yourself up. Understand that we are all really trying to do our best. Cultivate compassion toward yourself and others.

With consistency and perseverance, you will develop the necessary muscle. Then you will find yourself controlling your ego better, as well as understanding and embracing your own and others' flaws and shadows as part of our shared humanity. We realize what separates us is not knowledge or personal qualities but simply a confluence of personal circumstances. This will help you to continue making progress on your personal path to the truest and highest expression of yourself. We can only honor ourselves when we finally learn, honor, and understand our own flaws and shadows as part of the whole package.

We are all good and bad, tall and short, fat and thin, old and young, beautiful and ugly. One of the most potent self-realization moments I had in my life is when I realized that. During that time, I wrote this piece I am sharing with you now.

The Goodness

Goodness is pure,
but don't think it's unshakable,
because like all human emotion,
it is vulnerable...
It is fragile....
It is changeable!

Goodness is not constant.
It is not perfect.
It is a balance.

So, who are the good guys?
Do they exist? Where are they?
Would it be that the good ones are those who manage to develop a balance
between good and evil,
truth and lie,
innocence and lust?
Would it be that they are those who make peace with their demons,
who know them so well
that they know when to take them out for a walk and let them fly?

I certainly don't think they are the ones
Who tie and hide them in the closet as if they do not exist.
Those who bear themselves pure, virtuous, and unshakable,
to then martyr themselves inside,
tearing their hair out, to then
fail in their conquest of the impossible.

Let's face it, it's part of our nature
be sometimes good and sometimes bad.

Invite everyone to be kindest,
to make peace with their demons
and those of others.
I think that's the true
definition and the greatest test of goodness
and spiritual growth!

Don't shut them up.
Don't hide them.
Don't judge them.
Get to know them well,
and learn to live with them.
Since they—well balanced—
are an essential part of our talents and
those who open the doors to the unlimited potentials that we all have.

Time to make peace with our demons!

Ivel De Freitas, MD

If you want to dig more into this concept of living in nonduality, I recommend Dr. Shefali's book *A Radical Awakening,* where she explains how only by moving beyond duality are we able to release our shame and enter a real space of unconditional acceptance towards self and others.

I also want to invite you to check yourself on a compassion scale. So you can start developing awareness of areas that you need to work on. By developing self-compassion, life becomes more joyous, and accepting others' flaws becomes easier.

> "Self-compassion involves treating yourself with the same kindness, concern and support you'd show to a good friend."
>
> **—Kristin Neff**

Check the Kristin Neff self-compassion survey at www.self-compassion.org.

> "Our sorrows and wounds are only healed when we touch them with compassion."
>
> **—Buddha**

7. Cleanse your relationships.

Check your relationship often. Every single relationship has a level of toxicity. Ask the following questions of yourself:

- When you are together, does this person talk about himself or herself the whole time?
- Does he or she verbally put you or others down?
- Does the person make you feel guilty about the time you take for yourself?
- Do you feel burdened after spending time with him or her?

Take a moment to reflect on these questions. If you feel more miserable than happy when you spend time together, then you may need to set personal boundaries and take a step back from this person to protect yourself. Healthy boundaries are key to making any relationship sustainable. Boundaries allow a necessary space between you and the other person to allow room for individuality, self-love, and spiritual growth. Resist the natural temptation to break those boundaries.

Respect and foster healthy space between you and your loved ones. Include on this list not only your soulmate, but your children, family members, and friends. Do not sacrifice individuality for togetherness, thinking that this will help the relationship to mature and strengthen. When you love someone, it is natural to feel that you want to share and be a part of every single moment and event in the other one's life. But be aware that this is the most common mistake most of us make when we start a relationship. By suffocating your own and the other person's individuality, you are sentencing your relationship to death. The foundation of a positive and healthy relationship depends on maintaining and respecting individuals' differences. Protect your "ME space" and keep it clean, even when you have to force it. Go out with other friends even though you'd rather exclusively spend your time with this special person. I know it sounds weird, and the other person may not understand it either, but this is not selfish, but rather an act of self-love and love for the one you love.

You cannot love anyone fully and unconditionally without learning how to love yourself first. Space and boundaries help us in the process of getting there. They also foster better communication and tolerance for our differences. We are all interconnected, and although there are people who might make you feel special, happy, and loved, they do not deserve for you make them your main source of fulfillment and joy. Neither your partner, nor your children or friends deserve that. This sooner than later will become a "too much to bear" kind of situation, and you will end up burning each other out.

Don't fall for the delusion that comes from our own childish dream of loved ones are there to make us happy, so we don't have to do it ourselves. You and only you are the captain of your destiny and your emotions, the best healer for your own wounds and the best warrior for your own wars. You are your own savior, your best company, and your best partner in crime.

Once I realized this, I start treating myself better, lowered my expectations of others and becoming a better source on unconditional love for me and my family. I became a better partner, mother, daughter, friend, doctor, boss, and co-worker.

Here I share a piece I wrote in my journal while I was going through this process. This piece became my personal empowerment anthem. I invite you to try to write or find your own. Of course, if you like mine, you can use it too.

Yes, I Do!
Smells like a new life!
Smells like freedom!
Today is the first day I can fly...
Today I emerge from the cocoon...
With neither trauma nor noise,
as wanting no one to notice it,
so they don't spoil the moment.
And I smile, remembering that this is not possible anymore...
That this was part of my previous stage, of my prolonged childhood,
when I granted that power to others.
That was yesterday!

Today I spread my wings for the first time,
With great humility and infinite gratitude,
Today I remove my chains,
Chains I did not perceive and did not know even existed.
Chains I created to make me feel safe and secure.

But the universe drew me a plan and
aligned me with the masters and the moments,
the experiences and the lessons.
The universe tested me, and
I even dare to say...
On its leap of faith,
took a chance on me!

The truth is that I feel privileged,
For having understood the lessons and not letting me be
consumed by my fears and mundane feelings that threaten to
sabotage my process.

Today I surrender to my first flight
Filled with peace and confidence,
With no expectations, with no fear,
And I glide...
Surrendering with solemnity to this moment.
In blissful ignorance of my destiny...
Committed to honor the path wherever it takes me!

Today I fly with me!
Confident!
Without needing someone to hold a life net or show me the path!
And with this flight I start my adulthood,
I declare myself my ally forever!
I emancipate, fall in love, and get engaged with myself!
I marry me!
With my journey, my story,
My individuality,
My strength and my weakness,
My light and my shadows,
I marry my destiny whatever it is...
As long as it is with me!

Ivel De Freitas, MD

Love yourself!

We all know firsthand that life and relationships are not easy. We all have experienced challenging times. In fact, most experts in the field of personal development agree, the real work and the greatest opportunities to grow come with challenge, tragedy, and despair. Your work is to become your best ally, helping yourself to rebound, learn the lesson, move on, and proudly get back on track knowing yourself better. After all, the ultimate goal is to learn, grow, and thrive, becoming the highest, truest expression of yourself. That is what really sets you up to build better relationships based on trust, respect, empathy, and compassion. It allows you to better understand your and others' individual needs, making you a catalyst for joy and happiness. When you marry yourself and make peace with who you really are, with all your strengths and flaws on display, you will not only become a better person to relate with, but you will also attract like-minded people who will connect with you for who you really are. Have no shame. Be, love, and marry yourself.

Make Peace With Your Inner Self

> "Have you ever stood on the edge of the Grand Canyon, or gazed into the heavens by a calm lake on a moonless night? Did you feel yourself expand into that vast unimaginable vacuum, while at the very same instant you felt yourself collapse inward into your singleness, your simple insignificance? Is that a trick question? Maybe it only seems a little tricky because the answers to these crazy huge mysteries don't just lie out there in the infinite universal consciousness, but also right here, within the [not-so-finite] form that we call our Self."
>
> **—Robert Kopecky**

The most important relationship in life is the relationship you have with your inner self. Relationship with self is the foundation of everything else, health, happiness, performance, aging, and success.

Quoting one of my favorite paragraphs from the book *The Road Less Traveled* by M. Scott Peck:

> "Thus all life itself represents a risk, and the more lovingly we live our lives the more risks we take. Of the thousands, maybe even millions, of risks we can take in a lifetime the greatest is the risk of growing up. It is only when one has taken the leap into the unknown of total selfhood, psychological independence and unique individuality that one is free to proceed along still higher paths of spiritual growth and free to manifest love in the greatest dimensions."

Be your own best friend. Develop selfhood and embrace your traits as they are the foundation for your unique individuality.

However, you must remember that growing always takes time. And in this case, significant effort. To grow your inner self to the level of psychological freedom described by Scott Peck, you must work on it and make it one of your goals in life, otherwise it won't happen.

I am convinced that this is a key to achieving a life of fulfillment, as well as optimal health and aging beyond well.

A grownup inner-self allows you to be self-aware and cope well with your emotions, have clarity and a good sense of your values, and commit to a purpose. It also brings you the blessing of calmness, helping your ego to become more flexible, which helps you be less reactive. A flexible ego becomes your ally, allowing you to be more in control of your feelings and actions, so you act, instead of react, which as you know at this point it is key to keep your biology – including your cells and genes – and the inner chemistry – where your cells are embedded in – in better shape.

This is not easy, but it is definitely worthwhile. It is the only way to sustain the joy and happiness chemistry we want to cultivate to age beyond well. This is not just my opinion, but a consensus in the field of healthy longevity, epigenetics, positive psychology, and human development.

I have taken many journeys to my inner world. I usually start this journey by trying to find answers to why I have reacted or why I am feeling a certain way. Usually, I find the root to those reactions in my past, usually in my childhood. I can assure you—after spending most of my adult life studying this subject and using what I have learned in my medical practice—no one gets through childhood without some degree of wounding. No matter how great and loving your parents were, your unique individuality dictates how you will perceive and interpret any action they took. They are also human beings who have their own wounds and scars from their childhood. This, my friends, is present in any relationships we have and will impact the way what we say or do are perceived. If you stay blind to these facts, they have a way of subconsciously ruling you – body, mind, and genes included.

I will give you an example. I come from a household where my parents were very loving and at the same time very strict. My parents were on top of us. We had no free time to fool around. After I got married, I had to work on myself because I used to get upset and overreact whenever I felt my husband was trying to control me. Even his most innocent requests, such as call this person, do this, or move that, made me feel he was treating me like his assistant. I also used to resent his criticisms of my poor organization skills or juggling style of doing things.

I did not realize that I had the option of taking his comments as negative criticisms and feeling bad about it—or as opportunities to gain awareness and growth. I learned this when I tried to understand why his request or comments hurt me, when clearly he was not trying to. After working on it and analyzing the events, putting aside the emotional rush, I realized that these events were no more than a slight and gentle nudge from my husband for my own benefit. I became aware of the positive effect they could have on my own development, if I could learn to prevent my reactivity from blunting these special opportunities.

I started working on it. Even when the comments or requests sparked frustration or anger, if I was able to keep my mind clear, and act instead of react, the results were overall positive. They helped me to understand both our natures and look for ways to improve our communication and strengthen our relationship. Although sometimes difficult and painful, I started to appreciate these episodes and tried to perceive them more as opportunities for growth and learning and less as hurtful and bitter events. I compare these kinds of events to deep tissue massage. It hurts, but if you do not stop the process, in the end you'll see the benefits and feel better.

In this process of self-development, I start reading more about where these traits could be coming from. I learned how the dynamic with my parents was imprinted on my emotional makeup and made me react to things negatively that could be good for me overall. I also discovered that my natural rebel trait was coming from there and that this trait could be used for good or wasted on stupid and meaningless fights.

I learned that although relationships are one of the main culprits of conflict in our life, they are key in the process to achieve personal inner peace and aging beyond well. Once we discover that everyone is our *mirror* reflecting parts of our consciousness back *to* us, and the conflict they trigger is just pointing us hidden voids or gaps we all need to work on, we enable ourselves to grow and become more tolerant and even more appreciative of our differences. As our relationships with them improve, our relationship with ourselves follows and vice versa. Yes, your loved ones are there, as your mirrors and roadmaps, not as your transportation services, vehicles, fuel, salvation, or healers.

So, I trained myself to take my husband's inputs and requests as just opportunities to grow. I learned to choose which ones I'd take and which to ignore, instead of fighting or just being a good girl and trying to please him all the time, allowing me to honor and respect my individuality and autonomy. I also decided to put this natural rebel spirit to work for a good cause instead, becoming more aware of my emotions and connected with my self-development and growth. And this became one of my main sources of energy and passion.

Of course, it hasn't been easy. I have to exert a major amount of effort and discipline to prevent my natural instincts from taking over. This requires rewiring my brain to do what is really good for me and my own spiritual and professional development. When you find the scars from where your reactions come from, you start a healing process that leads you to real emotional freedom. It allows you to take control of your actions, and to make better and healthier choices.

I also chose to communicate my childhood hurts to my husband and with my children, dear friends, and family, so they could get to know me better and understand what triggers me and my reactions. Some people may feel this is too much, but that is me. I try to be an open book. I am proud of my vulnerability and my humanity. I have come to accept that we all have wounds and bruises, and I am convinced that when people love you they love you with those issues and not despite them. So, I have nothing to hide. In fact, I am proud of my capacity to recognize and carry my scars as little reminders that we are all humans, and we are not perfect. They are part of what defines and connects me with my peers, loved ones, and patients. They are part of who I am.

As I began accepting my weaknesses and flaws, I recognized I was more in control of my emotions. I recognized I could grow closer to the truest and highest expression of myself. I also grew more compassionate and understanding of myself and others. Compassion generates gratitude, and gratitude generates joy and resilience. This, my friends, is key to the quest for looking, acting, and feeling younger, the quest for healthy longevity and a life of fulfillment. It also helps to unleash new potential for changing the way your brain works. In my case, as I have been rewiring my brain and healing emotional wounds, I have become more creative. I even dare to write poetry. Here is another one of my creations:

Inner Journey

Few are the ones chosen for this journey...
Few are the ones who tolerate the noises of their own souls!
It is not easy to depart, but it is not easy to stay either...
And I remind you that despite you perhaps being chosen,
this does not make you better or worse.
Perhaps just a little weary, or maybe odd.
And definitely the ones who stay seem to be the normal ones.
And maybe they are.
But I can assure you that normal or not,
they are highly necessary.
They are our guides of the outer world.
They are the ones who help us to not get lost in our inner maze...
Because, despite being the ones who create many of our challenges
They also give us the reasons.
They are our mirrors constantly reminding us of who we are.
And they are the one who guide us on our way back.
Because what is it worth if you cannot share what you have learned and achieved with your loved ones?
With those who surround and support you, the one we call family, friends, and loved ones.
Because growth occurred traveling in the inner world and living in the outer world.
Today I come back from one of those inner trips empowered and awaiting my next journey.
Perhaps anxious to get started again but hesitant and a little fearful.
As these trips, despite hardships and many times painful,
always elevate me to a different dimension,
Destroying and rebuilding little by little
to become what I hope would be a more genuine and elevated expression of myself,
more authentic or perhaps just different!
Whichever ... is welcome!

Ivel De Freitas, MD

CHAPTER 8

GO

Once you have primed and reset your system, it is time to really biohack those genes to get what you want. However, to start getting what you want, you need first to define those specific goals in terms of your health and for your lifetime. To get what you want you need to first define exactly what it is you want, so you can start writing the script of your own story. This is key to bring you the benefits I want you to get. So, I encourage you to reflect on those areas you want to enhance and the goals you want to achieve. Think about those unique talents you possess and align them with your dreams, your highest desires. My goal is that through this process I can help you become the absolute best version of yourself. Empowering yourself holistically—mind, body, genes, and soul—can be transformative. But we have found that this process also helps to enhance your body's natural healing and rejuvenation powers.

Our body is meant to heal and stay healthy. Based on the science of peptides—short fragments of amino acids—normally produced by your body, this phase is founded on the belief that your natural healing and recovery powers can always be enhanced.

Peptides are key to repairing tissue and even gene alterations that may occur with aging, stress and chronic inflammation. Still under investigation, peptides' specific genetic activation powers are one of the most promising therapeutic tools under development and investigation today. I will first start by sharing simple strategies you can easily incorporate into your lifestyle that can help you enhance their natural production.

Fast for Your Life

Are you a breakfast person? Do you feel guilty when you skip breakfast? Is breakfast good or bad for you? Many of us grew up with parents fussing to make sure we had something in our bellies before we set off for school. We have also been brainwashed by the data supporting eating five small meals a day to keep our metabolism revving. Do you live by the motto that breakfast is the most important meal of the day? Have TV commercials' propaganda that promised eating cereal would make us lean and athletic influenced our natural behavior and shut down our intuition?

It turns out the research on eating breakfast has been far, far less conclusive than either your mother, physical trainer, dietitian school and Tony the Tiger would have you believe. In fact, if you've been eating breakfast to stave off weight gain, researchers are increasingly learning that breakfast might have the opposite effect—it can promote more calorie consumption and weight gain. But even the best available studies have serious limitations.

A recent scientific statement from the American Heart Association published in the journal *Circulation* noted that adults in the United States have moved from the traditional three meals a day schedule to eating around the clock.

Snacks, shakes, protein bars, and coffee breaks have become routine. As soon as the stomach is empty, there is food coming in again leaving no time for recovering and cleaning our poor gastrointestinal system. Bloating, constipation, and diarrhea have become major problems, and irritable bowel syndrome (IBS) is an epidemic.

In the meantime, what is happening in the blood and brain is even worse. This continuous food intake is a constant blood sugar level swing up and down that triggers insulin production continuously to compensate. As soon as blood sugar goes down, cravings and hunger start again, and people have something else to eat. This continuous food overflow overworks the pancreas—in part explaining the current epidemic of diabetes and obesity in America—and creates an unsustainable and undesirable blood sugar-insulin rollercoaster. This rollercoaster compromises an individual's energy, brain clarity, and mood in their day-to-day life, sabotaging their physical and mental performance and creating physical stress and inflammation.

The continuous presence of insulin in the blood also prevents human growth hormone (HGH) from spiking and doing its job. HGH has a key role in growth for children. It is also key to repairing cells, balances the metabolism, burns fat, and maintains healthy body composition in children and adults. It also boosts muscle growth, strength, and exercise performance, which are all key predictive markers for healthy longevity.

For all these effects, HGH has a positive reputation in the anti-aging medicine arena. We all produce it, and the most important spike happens at night.

Good sleep and fasting have been linked to increased HGH production. The elevated levels of HGH that you have at night are blunted as soon as insulin goes up when you eat in the morning. Studies have demonstrated that skipping breakfast and even exercising while fasting promotes fat burning, cellular regeneration, body rejuvenation, and even long telomeres and healthy longevity. Therefore, intermittent fasting (IF), which entails limiting the time during which food can be consumed on a given day, have gained popularity

While the molecular mechanisms have not been fully understood, there are evidence that supports this practice to prolong the life span, control blood pressure, and blood glucose levels. Furthermore, IF and calorie restriction were both shown to decrease the incidence of heart attack and stroke, as well as their ill effects. In particular, IF is thought to promote metabolic switching by altering gene expression profiles leading to reduced inflammation and oxidative stress, while increasing cellular plasticity and regeneration.

We have also learned autophagy, a cell-cleaning process, kicks in after fasting, but only when fasting occurs during the night. Autophagy (Greek for self-eating) is known to slow aging by cleaning up and recycling damaged components of the cell.

For all these reasons, I want you to consider skipping breakfast at least a few days of the week. In essence, our bodies function better—and we are healthier—when we press pause on eating for a stretch of time each day.

Although a growing body of evidence shows that certain forms of fasting might be good for you, I want to remind you that not everything is good for everyone. Personalization is the key to any plan. Although I suggest you give it a try and observe how you feel in terms of your energy and mood throughout the day when you skip breakfast, you need to take into consideration specific factors that might be important to decide if this would be good for you. For example, people who suffer from low blood sugar (hypoglycemia) and/or diabetes should work on their diet to normalize blood sugar and insulin levels with a specialist before embarking on something like skipping breakfast and experimenting with fasting strategies.

If you are one of those who force themselves to have breakfast because you have been told it is good for you, stop listening to everyone else and listen to your body.

If you have been eating breakfast all your life, cut down on the carbohydrates in the morning and try to have a protein breakfast instead of no breakfast at all. By cutting the carbs, you prevent insulin from rising, keeping your human growth hormone (HGH) higher for a longer time.

If you go to the gym in the morning and train for an hour or less you can try to continue fasting but remember to hydrate well with an unsweetened beverage or water. You can also have a branched-chain-amino acids (BCAA) or protein shake in the morning, as long as they do not have sugar or carbs.

Having unsweetened tea or coffee without sugar or milk won't break your fast either. You can have those during your fasting time and still get the benefits of a natural and spontaneous human growth hormone increase with the well-described anti-aging effect without the risk and inconvenience of using HGH replacement.

Stay Longer on GO Youth Mode: Break the Fast Right

It is important to remember that when you are skipping breakfast, eating healthy becomes imperative. If you want to fully enjoy the enhanced growth hormone effect that this strategic way of eating brings on, you need to fuel your body with the right nutrients when you break the fast. Although I still want you to eat what you want, I need you to pair that with nutritious food. So feed your soul with what you like and your core with what you need. As long as you keep that balance in mind, you will reap the benefits, positively impacting your health.

A nutritious diet reflects in your cellular and genetic makeup. It helps activate natural healing and enhance your immune system function, as well as stem cells and other natural regenerative powers. That's how diet can have an anti-aging and pro-longevity effect.

When you extend your fasting time by skipping breakfast, your immune system and stem cells work harder with this extra time for self-regeneration. Micronutrient, protein, amino acid, and antioxidant demand will ramp up. To keep the whole rejuvenation wheel rolling, you need to maximize your intake of macronutrients—especially proteins and healthy fats—and micronutrients—such as vitamins and minerals—and antioxidants during your eating periods.

As discussed in the first part of this book, your ideal meal plate should be half full of micronutrient- and antioxidant-rich food, which means half full of vegetables. The other half should be left for macronutrients like clean protein, healthy fat, and whole ancient grains. Remember that you are orchestrating all this around whatever you want and like to eat, keeping your promise of nourishing your core while nourishing your soul. (See illustration on page 121 to see again , what an ideal plate would look like).

Find What Sparks a Light in You, and Learn How to Light Up Your Genes Too

> "You often feel tired, not because you've done too much, but because you've done too little of what sparks a light in you."
>
> **—Alexander Den Heijer**

"Do what you love."

"Find your purpose."

"Follow your passion."

"Passion versus purpose."

"Purpose versus passion."

How in the hell do you find your passion and/or your purpose?

This debate has been going on for years.

Driven by fear of not being or having enough, we make it our life's mission to pursue wealth and fame, even when we are not passionate about the process.

That dream job, the one that you celebrated once, when you originally got it, progressively becomes an obligation, moving from something you wanted to do, to something you must do from paycheck to paycheck. How the heck did this happen?

We work more, play less, and neglect the very reason we strive for success in the first place: to grow as an individual, to share your unique talents, to contribute to society and to experience joy.

Joy never comes from having, but from sharing.

When what you wanted to do becomes a habit, and daily achievement becomes a routine, you get accustomed to your job. The exhilarating feeling of newness stops, and boredom replaces it. Fear also becomes a player—fear of staying stuck right where you are, fear of failure, fear of trying, fear of not being able to achieve fulfillment and joy again. At least that is how I once felt. When I was burned out.

When what you are giving is coming from a place of fear and scarcity you feel you are giving out what's left of you and you are expecting something in return, instead of when you are giving from a place of abundance and joy where giving become more an overflow. Where no effort is needed, and no expectations are held.

Living in place of scarcity and fear lead you to massive boredom, frustration and even anxiety and depression. Now we have added burnout to the labels we use to categorize this crisis. The difference is that one is treated with antidepressants and the other with a vacation or resignation and change of career. Both share feelings of despair, sadness, frustration, fear, and increased risk of suicide.

When you are burned out, you feel you have lost control of your destiny. You feel you are sacrificing, you are stretching your will and continuing because you have no other option. When you feel life has taken over, it is frustrating, frightening, and, in fact, paralyzing.

So, when your day-to-day actions and reactions come from fear, you feel overwhelmed and defeated. You feel you have no control. You feel like a puppet. This has a negative impact on your body and your biomolecular core. It also creates a vicious cycle that kidnaps your mind and inner self and sabotages your way out. It disrupts balance, saps creativity and energy, and neutralizes your attempt to reclaim your personal passion. It affects productivity, morale, and even how you interact with others—all while robbing you of time and happiness. It eclipses the joy of working with a sense of obligation, self-sacrifice, and lack of control.

Have you felt like that? These feelings can originate in any area of your life, from your professional role, to your role as parent, partner, a devoted adult child or sibling, and romantic lover.

After many years of painful emotional falls and laborious bounces back, one of the most important strategies I have learned to minimize my self-doubt, despair, and self-defeating moments is to take the focus off myself and my despair and shift my focus to others. When you take away the focus off yourself and on to others, you realize that other people have problems, too. In fact, you may have ways to help them find their way out. This is one of the multiple valuable lessons I learned from *The Book of Joy*. The book narrates the last meeting of His Holiness Dalai Lama and Desmond Tutu when they were together to celebrate the eightieth birthday of the Dalai Lama. During that meeting they sat and shared their thoughts and experiences, giving us the best gift they could have ever given to humanity, sharing their own experiences and strategies to foster joy in their life. This book has been so helpful on my spiritual journey that it is one of the books that I permanently keep on my bedside table and grab any time my soul is invaded by self-doubt, fear, and despair.

Nonetheless, I have to say that as time has passed, although I still have moments of failure and despair, I have realized something that is key to the process of making the dark moments shorter.

I have gotten better at retraining my brain, just as these two holy spiritual leaders have mastered throughout their lives. And although I'm far from that kind of magnificent and unprecedented spiritual wisdom, I keep getting better at mastering my own strategies. I celebrate every time I bounce back, and I recognize that I get stronger and wiser with each crisis. And, although I don't celebrate them when they arrive—I celebrate them when I overcome them.

Another empowering strategy is to face these moments with the right attitude. Treat these moments as opportunities to grow and evolve, lessons that will help you to reshape and restore your ways and attitudes. They are a kind of foundation checkpoint or maintenance protocol.

This thinking process will refocus your attention on others and recognize them as opportunities to grow. They also give you the opportunity to find purpose in your difficulties, pain, or suffering. Finding a purpose in your worst moments and experiences not only brings hope to you during these moments—"this too shall pass"—but has become instrumental in my own and many of my patients' processes for building a life of happiness and fulfillment. These experiences have convinced me that this is an essential formula you should use to allow you to stay in love with your life, your job, your roles, and your story—to achieve your highest potential and age beyond well.

Stay in Love to Keep You Going!

Life is easier when you are in love, don't you agree? I am not necessarily talking here about being in love with your partner though. I refer to being in love with your reality. I mean your life, your work, your mission, your passion, your talents, your flaws, your story, and your loved ones.

As anything in life, in order to stay in love and make the honeymoon period last a lifetime you need to invest energy and time in it. This kind of blessing doesn't happen accidentally. It is a decision you have to make and a lifetime mission you need to commit to.

At any given time, you are either consciously choosing to prove that love can last forever or not. This decision depends on what you choose to focus on.

If you choose to focus on the positive and the blessing of each and every moment, and stay open to learning, perceiving life as an adventure, letting go of control of what you cannot control, you are buying a ticket to nirvana.

Newness and gratitude are key parts of the formula. Without adventure and newness, the honeymoon ends quickly and sadly for any relationship, including the relationship you have with your profession and with yourself.

This mindset is something you need to create. It is not natural for human beings to focus on their blessings. Instead, they tend to focus on their shortcomings.

For centuries humanity has been able to survive thanks to the capacity to focus on upcoming problems—it allowed people to prepare for winter and trying times. This is wired deeply in our brains, printed in our genetic blueprint.

To be positive and grateful, you need to retrain and rewire your brain purposefully. It takes time and repetition to create this habit, like any other habit. And even when you think you have it all figured out and you mastered the nirvana-honeymoon mindset, suddenly life hits you and you fall again, hitting the ground filled with self-doubt. I have been there and done that, just like any other person who is trying to master this mindset.

In the Quest

Do not look any further
Don't torment yourself
Relax, breathe...
Connect.
Listen, understand!

What you are looking for so much
It is there, in your space
in your process.
It is there, in their space
in their process.
But above all, it is there
in that magical and intimate space,
shared by souls
living and sharing
the everyday.

As in any interaction with someone new,
initially the novelty for whatever you are doing
let the fascination come easy,
It is there in anything you see
In anything that keeps you busy.
But the novelty doesn't last forever
No matter what we do
Or what you say.
Everyday life arrives!
And with it, new challenges,
But also new colors, new nuances, new rhythms, and
sometimes new forces.
But not everyone can see
the beauty, the pure, the sexy; in the peace and quietness of
everyday life, and
so, they flee to the new,
missing the opportunity to experience the fascinating
spectrum of sensations,

learning, moments that everyday life has to offer.
A spectrum that leads
to the highest levels of joy,
of love, satisfaction, and peace.

But to get there you have to get out of the box
where everything looks the way you like it,
And take on the task of understanding the hidden world
held inside of you and the other who are living with you.
A world to be explored with the eyes of a traveler,
the soul of a child,
the flexibility of a contortionist,
the tenacity of marathonist,
the adaptability of a salamander, and
the enthusiasm of a new lover.

Just fascinating for those of us who give ourselves to the task
to learn how to discover them.

I confess, it is not an easy adventure,
It requires a lot of growth,
A lot of interior cleaning
Much patience
And above all a lot of expansion
Beyond what one believes,
of what one sees.
Beyond yourself and your ego!
But of one thing there is no doubt,
it is worth the effort!

And so,
What do we do when everyday life arrives?
Let us cultivate it, celebrate it, and embrace it, as the greatest of treasures of all,
because in the climax of everyday life is where the maximum degree of well-being,
love and happiness is reached,
The place where we become the best expression of ourselves,
transcending the borders of our limited humanity,
integrating with each other in true unity.
Where we experience oneness!

Ivel De Freitas, MD

Life is ephemeral, so we had better enjoy it. Living to the fullest is all about balance. Friends and family gatherings, social events and laughing, especially laughing out loud (LOL), is as beneficial for your biomolecular core and telomeres as sleeping eight hours, exercising, stretching your growth hormone curve, and eating adequate amounts of antioxidants and micronutrients. Consequently, if you want to be successful and max out your chance to turn back your clock, unlock your highest genetic potential and fulfill your dream of a happy and healthy long life, you need to give yourself permission to enjoy things, in the most organic and natural fashion you can.

This, my friends, is key to keeping your telomeres long and your life fulfilled. And it will also make the journey worthwhile and allow you to finally achieve what we all want in life. As brilliantly expressed by Oprah Winfrey, to become the truest highest expression of oneself, you must enjoy the path!

Monitoring Your Body Clock

Controlling your body clock may sound like something out of a science fiction film, but you really could be getting younger this year. Of course, I am not talking about your chronological age but your "biological age."

After all, isn't that what really matters?

Of course, monitoring your body clock requires you to commit to taking control over your aging process and make the adjustments necessary in your diet, supplementation, and lifestyle.

At this point, I hope you already have a very good understanding that the foundation of your health, quality of life and longevity lies in your biomolecular core. So, everything we have mentioned in the two steps discussed are determinants for how fast you age, and for how good you look, act, and feel.

To get on the road of turning back your body clock, you need to first recognize and honor your unique biomolecular individuality, which means that your needs are different from the needs of other people and that you must meet them in order to fulfill your own highest potential and optimize your longevity and quality of life.

Going to the vitamin shop or buying whatever is being offered on the Internet as the panacea for whatever complaint you may have is no longer okay for you. You have come a long way and educated yourself enough to understand that your needs are no longer the same as everyone else's. Whatever the vitamin shop guy or personal trainer is telling you to buy or take in terms of supplements and vitamins is no longer good enough for you; without knowing your unique biomolecular values and profile, these recommendations are useless.

My research and the work of many others in the field support that by providing the right nutrient at the right time to the right individual, we can gain control of our biological clock—not only slowing down the process but even turning it back.

The very first thing you need to do to get on this plan is to calculate your current biological age.

To do that, you can use any of the tools currently available for you to monitor your BioAge.

I have created one that I use with my patients, and you can access it for free at ONOGEN.com. This tool is designed to determine your BioAge based on your lifestyle.

The second way to learn more about your biological age is testing your telomeres and epigenetic age. I recommend using truage.com for your epigenetic age or lifelength.com, spectracell.com or cellsciencesystem.com for your telomeres as those are the one I have chosen to use in my clinical practice.

I recommend these tests to be done once per year to monitor pace of aging and telomeres and epigenetic DNA changes. Analyzing this data helps us *to* gauge *the* effectiveness of your lifestyle efforts and adjust your plan accordingly. Don't you want to be sure that your lifestyle strategies are worth the effort or if something needs to be changed?

All the steps I am giving you here are aimed at getting you to live younger longer, which means living, feeling, acting, and looking younger. All my recommendations are based on real scientific evidence. Your job is to follow these steps and to fine-tune them specifically for you.

PART III

THE FUTURE

CHAPTER 9

A New Era Has Begun

Ever since Steve Jobs put the Internet in everyone's pocket, our lives have been utterly transformed, marking the beginning of a new era. Since then, the world has reorganized itself around smartphone technology. But the iPhone effect goes far beyond smartphones.

The Internet initially brought us multiple advantages: allowing people to access information and even shop from the convenience of their own house or office. Smartphones have brought us to a futuristic dimension, where anything seems possible and achievable, as long as you have your smartphone with you. This changed our relationship with technology way beyond "convenience" to "lifeline."

Do you remember those days when getting a cab was a stroke of luck, especially if you were on a side street, or coming out of a late dinner in the middle of the night? The fact that we are now able to get a ride with just a little swipe from wherever we are to wherever we want, at any time, is scarcely believable. But wait, it gets better! This technology also gives you the option to choose the type and size of car and even the personality trait of the driver you are getting. If you are not in the mood for a chatty driver, you just check the reviews and get one who is described as polite and quiet.

Now the concerns are over what we are losing or giving up in return. While people are spending more time heads down, buried in their phone, we are also becoming accustomed to a new sense of stress. Too much is going on at the same time, so much that it is almost impossible to get away from even if you want to. Your clients, friends, and partners now expect a reply from a text message as soon as they send it. You are supposed to always be connected—always available, always ready to reply from wherever you are at whatever time it is.

But like it or not, this revolution has taken over! Perhaps it is more an evolution than a revolution. Despite concerns that the enchanting effects of technology are taking away our freedom and moving us from the real world to a virtual world, smartphones have still become our most resourceful and unconditional companion, transforming every single area of our lives. Education, photography, music, communication, politics, advertising, finances, banking, commerce, parenthood, marriage, and even dating have been impacted and changed forever. And with that, the bar of consumers' expectations has been raised to levels we never thought possible.

Meanwhile, when COVID-19 hit, it reframed even more the consumers' health needs, motivation, and priorities. Health has become wealth, while wellness and self-care have become priorities.

Simultaneously, biohacking—defined as the use of technology and science to self-enhance health and well-being—emerged as a trend that rapidly became a collective potential disruptor for healthcare.

As new ideas are sourced online, anyone with an interest in self-care becomes a biohacker, and biohacking becomes the new self-care. Biohacking is no longer a trend. It is self-care 2.0, a shift in patients' mentality that demands a change in healthcare.

Electronic medical records and robotic surgery are now standard at hospitals and medical offices, telemedicine continues to rise at exponential rates, and iPhone and smartphone apps are advancing biometrics to help patients track important health markers. Meanwhile, doctor-patient relationships struggle to adjust to this new era. As patients want to team up and make their own health decisions based on their intuition and preference instead of passively accepting whatever the insurance company approves for them or the doctor in front of them advises, doctors are trying to cope with this new demand in a system that is not built to support that.

THE INDUSTRY TRANSFORMATION

Consumerization in Healthcare

"Patients are now consumers who have power, choices and opinions about their care. They want an experience that is convenient and seamless, while also being personalized."

Forbes

QUOTE: Forbes https://www.forbes.com/sites/blakemorgan/2020/10/01/post-covid-19-patient-experience-3-ways-healthcare-has-changed/#602086b5b59f

This sudden rise in expectations has also imposed a new challenge on a relationship that was already struggling, forcing a change in the dynamic of the doctor-patient relationship and disrupting the status quo.

As a response, the status quo in medicine is shifting, as it's obvious that the current medical model and healthcare paradigm is failing to meet the needs of a new era of "health literacy," biohackers, and empowered users.

Nanotechnology, gene therapy, biohacking, life extension, healthy longevity, singularity, immortality! Buzzwords that are defining the beginning of this new era in healthcare. But how long can we really live? And how good can those years potentially be?

Dramatic breakthroughs in medicine and public health have resulted in unprecedented extensions of the human lifespan. However, on the quest of redefining aging and longevity, the collective longing is not really for more years but for better quality.

A life where aging may not mean losing vitality and functionality physically, mentally, and emotionally but maintaining or even gaining it. A life that is not simply longer, but healthy and happy, allowing each individual to become the absolute best version of her/him/themself.

I have made it my mission to collaborate in the creation of a new foundation for renovating healthcare and the existing medical model. I am convinced that by embracing the collective biohacking movement, we are literally supporting the shift of our current outdated model toward a more participative, equalitarian, and inclusive healthcare system.

In this approach, the individual's participation channeled through an innovative and intuitive biohacking model is key. I envision this as a movement that champions patient preference, intuition, and values as being equal to medical expertise.

The Biohacking Revolution

Biohacking is one of the most significant collective breakthroughs in the health industry of the twenty-first century. It is a gentle, changing force, a silent healthcare revolution, which is pushing for progress and change. A silent revolution that is slowly demanding easy access to the latest innovations in biotechnology and medicine, testing the system at a level that has never been tested before.

While the advertising and e-commerce industry are creating campaigns to sell products and services to fulfill the new demands of these health-literate consumers, topics like "right to try" (allowing the use of experimental therapies in cases of serious or life-threatening illnesses) have invaded Congress, and biology, genes, biochemistry, and biomolecular terms are slowly becoming less abstract and complex for everyday users.

Consumers now recognize that understanding their personal biological makeup may allow them to more wisely choose the best diet, exercise, and even medical therapy to enhance their body and mind and to activate natural healing. They are now more than ever willing to try new, innovative technology to enhance and optimize their overall health, wellness, and longevity.

Biohacking has patients moving from passive users to proactive searchers of the latest and the best. Doctor-patient relationships are now being pushed to move to real partnerships where both parties bring their wisdom to the healthcare decision-making process. We should all be excited, as this represents a new era where our job is more important than ever because the consumer is obtaining information from reliable and unreliable sources. As providers our job is to raise the bar and understand that our responsibility is not to know everything, which has become impossible, but to become the compass that helps patients navigate and translate the vast amount of information that exists out there.

Patients are more participative in their healthcare than ever before, but the system is not ready for it. The time we get per encounter is not designed for this kind of consultation and is not reimbursed for it either. We are talking about a consultation that needs more talking, education, and negotiation than just a quick assessment, diagnosis, and writing a script.

Not surprisingly the system is failing. It needs to change to a real shared decision-making (SDM) dynamic model, where patients and clinicians have an open discussion about the current trends and the best available evidence, and each decision or choice about health (tests, procedures, treatment, behaviors) is made balancing risk and expected outcomes with patient preferences and values. For this to happen, insurance companies' reimbursement systems need to change to recognize and reimburse the time and effort and respect and cover the decision made.

But patients and providers also need to change. We need to make peace with each other and team up collectively because our future depends on it. If COVID-19 has not served as a wakeup call, I don't know what else we need.

From Reactive to Proactive

Although medicine has existed since the beginning of humanity, with the goal of solving the problem of illness, it is time to recognize that this primitive reactive model does not serve us anymore. New and proactive health markers need to emerge to couple with technological advancements, beyond electronic medical records and access portals for patients to see their tests.

Why are we waiting for a problem to appear when it should be proactively prevented? With the confluence of medicine and technology, the finalization of the human genome project, and progress in the overlapping fields of robotics, artificial intelligence, gene therapy, nanotechnology, and functional and regenerative medicine, people's needs and expectations deserve to be met.

Changes to well-established and specialized complex structures are always more challenging. To make this strong and rigid structure adapt to what is coming, the reorganization of the system needs to begin by revising its foundation first.

Breakthroughs in medicine, public health, and social and economic development have come a long, long way, resulting in unprecedented extension of life expectancy, from about fifty years in the year 1900 to about seventy-three years in 2022. This demographic shift has imposed new challenges to the modern healthcare system—those additional years seem to be burdened with chronic diseases that the system can barely manage. It cannot cure them, which is compromising the sustainability of the system itself. Sixty percent of people above sixty-three years of age suffer from two or more chronic conditions. Novel strategies are urgently needed to transform the way we age and maximize the number of years lived in good health. We need to ensure better health, functional capacity, quality of life, well-being, and productivity during a period of extended longevity. The time has arrived to challenge the status quo and medicine's foundation to be rethought and reshaped to better serve us.

The clamor for better health options, prompted by the aging of the baby boomers, can no longer be ignored. We all want to age beyond well. TIME magazine's cover consistently features health topics such as "Why Your DNA Isn't Your Destiny," "This Baby Could Live To Be 142 Years Old," and "2045: The Year Man Becomes Immortal," and similar articles flood the Internet, the news, and newspapers. Anti-aging medicine has moved beyond Botox and aesthetics to genetics, exosomes and stem cells. Numerous direct-to-consumer genetics-related health companies, such as 23andMe and Eone Diagnomics Genome Center (EDGC) have emerged to meet this interest in a more proactive, preventive, personalized, and participative approach to medicine with the ultimate goal of healthy longevity.

Personalized Medicine, an Unstoppable Revolution

Recognition that physicians need to take individual variability into account has played a role in this rise of media interest in a new healthcare industry trend. Since 2015, when President Barack Obama announced a $215 million national Precision Medicine Initiative, which includes among other things, the establishment of a national database of genetic and other data of one million people in the United States, the industry has reacted accordingly.

Numerous pharmaceutical and technology companies are investing in making medicine more precise and personalized, initiating the era of personalized medicine. This includes a common goal of improving optimal longevity that takes in consideration not only lifespan but healthspan.

Different terms have emerged to describe this new area, such as "personalized medicine," "precision medicine," "genetic medicine," and "personalized genomics." They are all used to describe a range of genetics-related healthcare practices through which we define patients' bioindividuality. Bioindividuality is the myriad factors—medical, biomolecular, genetic, and environmental, among others—that shape a person's health, longevity, and response to a particular treatment. "Personalized medicine" and "precision medicine" have become the most popular concepts. And while people try to define each one of them, there is still a lack of consensus on their definitions. What is widely accepted is that precision medicine incorporates the concept of bioindividuality to create groups of similar people to develop a more targeted approach toward their shared similarities. "Personalized medicine," on the other hand, has been avoided for most groups because it implies that treatments and preventive strategies are being developed uniquely for each individual. Which, in my opinion, is exactly what our ultimate goal should be.

As I see it, precision medicine encompasses just the first baby steps to get medicine and technology to change and evolve toward an advanced personalized approach. This would bring us to create therapy based on a more functional concept of bioindividuality, a concept that I like to call Bioindividuality 2.0.

From "One-Size-Fits-All" to Bioindividuality 2.0

Nevertheless, although the status quo "one-size-fits-all" approach to medicine is being challenged, most treatment plans are still delivered based on what we learned in the second half of the twentieth century, from the "Antibiotic Revolution."

Before antibiotics were available, most diseases were regarded as a self-limiting, inconvenient illness caused by changes in the environment and susceptibility of the patient. Since the discovery of penicillin, followed by the development of other antimicrobials, that approach changed radically. Please do not misunderstand me. I recognize that Fleming's discovery of penicillin in 1928 is one of the major breakthroughs in medicine, changing the way doctors treated patients with infectious diseases and contributing to the control of infectious diseases that were the leading causes of human morbidity and mortality for most of human existence.

However, the antibiotics era also initiated and established a model and status quo that no longer serves us. A model founded on finding the diagnosis and killing or poisoning the disease with a drug-of-choice model. Treating under this model all kind of ailments from headaches to cancer.

Therefore, instead of supporting the body's natural healing mechanism, we became enchanted with the idea of being more efficient and effective. "Let's just kill the bugs" became our new motto, as well as the source of new problems. We left behind the most important factors that determine outcome—the patient and his or her own bioindividuality. When we treat the patient as a secondary factor, we tend to discriminate against the development of simpler and more beneficial "common sense" interventions, those that enhance the natural immune defenses and healing powers, such as micronutrient intravenous therapy, the Myers' Cocktail, peptides, diet, lifestyle modification, and meditation. They have all been called complementary and alternative, when in fact they should have been integrated into the mainstream long ago.

Our therapeutic strategies became more focused on drugs and procedures to cure the disease, kill the bug, eradicate the cancer, and eliminate risk factors such as cholesterol and blood sugar, than on the imbalances that originally caused the problem. This led to a narrow and fragmented, "one-size-fits-all" therapeutic model that is becoming obsolete and even absurd. Trying to treat chronic diseases and other life-threatening health challenges like cancer, where the traditional approach of solving the problem by killing it with drugs or removing it with surgery is no longer efficient and effective enough. Better strategies are needed to get better outcomes. Healthcare needs a more preventive and proactive approach to really impact the epidemic of preventable lifestyle- and aging-related chronic conditions, like heart disease, hypertension, type 2 diabetes, and undesirable treatment-related complications.

The patient's own natural healing systems need to be considered every time we are facing a new problem—even our grandma knew that! It is time for this old school diagnosis-centered and reactive approach to be replaced by a more sensitive, proactive, personalized, and efficient approach. These are the reasons why a personalized, predictive, proactive, preventive, and participative medicine is more than welcome now to fill the gaps created by a system that is longing for change.

Bioindividuality 2.0: Are We There Yet?

The idea of individualism has been getting stronger within Western societies over the last two centuries. Although the concept was initially used for its moral and social connotation that advocated the rights for freedom and self-realization of the individual, it evolved with the mapping of the human genome, incorporating the biomolecular factor into the equation.

While mankind's genetic make-up is 99.1 percent identical, a small 0.9% inter-individual, genetic differences explain the vast variability that exists within the human species. The need to celebrate an individual's uniqueness goes beyond a cultural trend on social media, TV, movies, and press to an opportunity to make medicine break its own paradigms.

Moving medicine approaches from broad therapeutic strategies to a heterogeneous population to a unique treatment approach based on a patient's bioindividuality should become our new paradigm. Happily, we are witnessing the first steps of this with the beginning of biomolecular medicine and a more targeted approach to cancer.

With the development of specific cancer therapies targeting an individual tumor's genetic markers, scientists have now moved to incorporate the patient's genes into the diagnostic and treatment paradigm. This means they not only focus on cancer genes, but also on the genes of the patient who is getting the therapy—genes that can determine adverse reactions and side effects. This opens possibilities for assigning therapy by the diagnosis, as well as by the patient's bioindividuality.

Incorporating this concept can be used to better obtain a positive outcome, and to decrease the chance of adverse side effects. It is forcing scientists and physicians to rethink the foundations of our current model, opening opportunities for new therapies to emerge, such as immunotherapies and cellular therapies that aim to boost the body's natural defenses and healing mechanisms—to fight cancer, accelerate healing, or even enhance human capacities and longevity. It is about time that our therapeutic plans start focusing on more than toxic drugs that kill the bug or the cancer, but in many cases weaken the patient's natural healing mechanism. As the old saying goes, "The cure is worse than the disease."

A great example of how this concept is infiltrating slowly into medicine is thymosin alpha 1. This is an immunomodulatory peptide with a natural anti-viral activity that has been found to boost the number and activity of a subset of immune cells in charge of killing viruses and cancer. This peptide is naturally produced by the thymus in humans. Production of peptides decrease as the thymus shrinks and its function decreases with aging. After multiple studies demonstrating its positive effect controlling liver cancer related to hepatitis B and C and melanoma with minimal side effect profiling, the drug was approved by the FDA to be used for this subset of patients.

Thymosin alpha 1 (thymalfasin, its pharmaceutical form) is also now indicated as a adjuvant therapy for chemotherapy-induced immune depression, immune insufficiency, and immune suppression in patients with non-small cell lung carcinoma (NSCLC), malignant melanoma, hepatocellular carcinoma (HCC), breast cancer, non-Hodgkin's lymphoma (CHOP program), colorectal cancer, head and neck cancer, leukemias, pancreatic carcinoma, and renal cell carcinoma. Clinical studies in over 1000 patients with various types of cancer demonstrated that thymosin alpha 1 improved immunological parameters, increased tumor response rates, and improved survival and quality of life. Thymosin alpha 1 was either administered for six months or given between chemotherapy cycles for the duration of treatment. Although, for many years, we have been using agents to reestablish immunity in between chemotherapies, such agents did not influence the tumor response rate because they worked by increasing white blood cells, with no proven effect on the specific subset of cells (natural killer cell, NK) that thymosin alpha might hold.

This is just the beginning, thymosin alpha is also being actively studied and showing results in the management of COVID-19, decreasing risks of complications and mortality. There are also studies that support its use as a vaccine effect enhancer. This is something that I have been bringing up since the beginning of the pandemic, as I have been following the data and have been passionate about peptides for many years.

However, all these studies are being done abroad because thymosin alpha 1 that was available in the United States through some compounding pharmacies, has been recently banned from the market and some of us are working on supporting the reestablishment and the continuation of the research. Although a setback, the revolution will continue. Progress is not progress without deviation of the norm, challenging of the status quo, and insistence on reform. The revolution must go on until balance is reached.

> "Beyond our idea of wrong-doing and right-doing, there is a field. I will meet you there."
>
> —Rumi

This revolution mode, calmly and consciously, should also be brought to our primary care offices and hospital bedside, breaking the current status quo with friendly technology that not only makes paperwork and rule compliance easier as it is now, but Bioindividuality 2.0 more achievable.

The "killing-the-bug" approach has kept our medical system reactive, marginalizing prevention and proactive care. It has left us with tools that only allow us to diagnose illnesses and diseases, pairing prevention with early diagnosis, which means that most efforts are directed toward detecting the disease early in its course. Instead of preventing it in the first place to develop.

Scientists are trying to group people by their bioindividuality to create a new path for medicine. Most of what they are focusing on at the molecular level is your genetic blueprint, which represents, in my opinion, the main flaw of this emerging new model. Although it remains true that your DNA—your genetic code—provides the blueprint for your biological and molecular makeup, the field of epigenetics now recognizes your genes are more a prediction than a life sentence. Whatever is written in your genes is not necessarily what is currently happening with you at the molecular level, which is what really defines your bioindividuality.

In other words, what is written in your genes is another determinant of what is happening inside your biomolecular core, but it does not represent a picture of all that is currently happening there. It is more like a prediction, telling us the odds of having or developing certain deficiencies, but not necessarily the presence of them at the specific time of examination or evaluation.

Despite, the use of some functional markers available today, I have been using to formulate therapies for my patients. There is no doubt that better markers need to be developed to give a better, more accurate, and functional reflection of an individual's bimolecular core—Bioindividuality 2.0. I hope my work and the work of others pioneering this field can contribute to the development of these kinds of functional and dynamic markers.

> "If there is no struggle, there is no progress."
> **—Frederick Douglass**

I am convinced that things will change for the better, and that soon the trend of personalizing nutrients based on genetic profiles will evolve to a real personalization based on dynamic and functional testing and evidence-based protocols.

This is a very exciting moment to be a doctor. We are at an inflection point in medicine. We are witnessing a renaissance that will change the way we care for people. Empowering concepts such as bioindividuality and the biomolecular core, and the technological growth and advancement in artificial intelligence (AI) and regenerative medicine are forces that are driving the current medical model toward a more personalized, proactive and patient-centered model.

> "It is far more important to know what person the disease has than what disease the person has."
> **—Hippocrates**

Meanwhile, we still have many paradigms to break and work to do. A great example is what the traditional approach has done with risk factors, the closest markers we have to an early and more proactive approach. Today, risk factors are approached as diagnosis, which means they are treated with drugs and sometimes surgery. This is more proof that even though our diagnostic and therapeutic tools are advanced, our approach and model are still primitive.

I watch with horror how new genetic advancements are incorporated into the system, as yet another diagnosis to be treated, adhering to a standard of care predetermined by an obsolete model. Here's an example: how traditional medicine approaches *BRCA* genes. The *BRCA1* and *BRCA2* genes are two of the most common genes known to be associated with an increased risk of cancer, most notably breast and ovarian cancer. Everyone has *BRCA1* and *BRCA2* genes, but some people, 1 in 400, may carry a mutation in one or both of these genes. When there is a mutation in one or both, DNA repair mechanisms may no longer be effective, which increases the risk of cancer, breast, ovarian, and pancreatic cancer for women and prostate, pancreatic, and breast cancer for men.

The risk of breast cancer for the average American woman is about 12 percent in her lifetime. The estimated risk of breast cancer in women with a BRCA mutation is 45 to 85 percent by age seventy years, depending on multiple factors.

Traditional medicine recommends an approach that goes from having a bilateral mastectomy to frequent testing and surveillance, exposing this patient to significant amounts of radiation which might itself increase their risk of mutations and cancer. However, not everyone who has the gene develops the disease. Environment, lifestyle, stress, and emotional factors have all been linked to breast cancer as well, although that is somewhat disregarded by the current standard approach as there is not designed intervention to address these areas on these patients. Don't you agree that proposed interventions should be built in a more holistic and integrative model? While new gene therapies are being developed to repair or counteract mutated genes, and precision medicine continues trying to determine which group of patients should be treated more aggressively, the best is yet to come. But we need to be patient and exercise caution. Although this science is in development, current advances should not be underestimated. If you or any of your loved ones are going through a similar challenge, make sure you explore all the possibilities before committing to an aggressive approach. Trust your intuition, educate yourself and make an informed decision, don't just do what your friend or doctor tells you. Yes, I am a doctor, and I am saying that. For these kinds of decisions, you get second and even third opinions, even if you are seeing me this is what I will tell you.

Singularity: Can We Live Forever?

In 2015 according to WHO, global life expectancy at birth averaged 69 to 73 years, with females living longer than males. However, people say, oh, I don't want to live past 90 but you know, I talk to 90-year-olds, and they want to live to 91 and even to 100. People sometimes say that death gives meaning to life because it makes time more valuable.

From the voice of Jane Fonda on a TED Talk she did, that I highly recommend you watch, where she divides life into three stages of thirty years, calling the one she is in the Third Act. "But now that I am actually smack-dab in the middle of my own third act, I realize I've never been happier. I have such a powerful feeling of well-being. And I've discovered that when you're inside oldness, as opposed to looking at it from the outside, fear subsides. You realize you're still yourself—maybe even more so."

At the increasing pace of progress, we are on our way to soon being able to overcome many diseases and even aging. Futurist visionaries like Ray Kurzweil, Google's chief futurist – author of *Singularity is Near* and *The Age of Spiritual Machines* – dare to challenge mortality, becoming one of the biggest believers in "the singularity." Thanks to him and other scientists, the singularity is becoming a movement that believes that at some point humans—with the aid of technology—will live forever. This hypothetical point in time described an uncontrollable and irreversible technological growth that will result in unforeseeable changes to human civilization. In his book, *The Singularity is Near*, he predicts that singularity will be achieved by the year 2045. He predicts singularity will render human immortal, recreating your humanity using technology, backing up most of our thinking in a non-biological form to be able to live indefinitely. Based on his calculations, by that time, non-biological intelligence will reach a level that is a billion times more powerful than all human intelligence today. He also predicts that this will occur and increase exponentially, not incrementally or following a linear pattern of growth. So, by the year 2029, medical technology will be able to add one additional year every year to your remaining life as per his calculations. He explained that after the year 2029, medical technology should begin to fix some of the underlying biological causes of aging, allowing this natural limit to be surpassed, adding extra years to your personal lifespan. Finally, computers will become so powerful that they can model human consciousness. This will permit us to download our personalities into non-biological substrates. When we cross this bridge, we become information, and then, if we maintain multiple copies of ourselves to protect against a system crash, we won't die.

He encourages everyone to make their best effort to get there alive by using aggressive lifestyle and antiaging therapies.

Whether we agree with the concept of singularity, the overlapping revolutions of human genetics, artificial intelligence, and nanotechnology are going to exponentially transform not only healthcare, but as he specifically predicts in his book, every institution and aspect of human life, from sexuality to spirituality. This transformation promises to enhance individual human capabilities, and radically upgrade human physical and mental capacities. I have embraced the same goal not only in my personal life, but also in my medical practice—moving from the standard state of "well enough" to *beyond well*. Isn't this what all physicians and patients should be striving for?

However, to change the model, technological progress and effort should be redirected, incorporating dynamic concepts, such as functional biomolecular deficiencies, stem cell functionality and immunity and biological age to recreate the foundation of medicine. Embracing markers that better reflect Bioindividuality 2.0, prioritizing the achievement of biomolecular harmony to optimize natural regeneration, immunity, and healing pathways, aiming to improve therapeutic outcomes. To achieve this, we need to prioritize our health and be more proactive in developing our own personal formula for success. Becoming our best self-advocates, biohacking our health, longevity, and happiness.

CHAPTER 10

The Four Pillars of Future Medicine

Entertaining the idea of reshaping medicine represents one of the most exciting challenges that all this revolution imposes on us. As we recognize that moving medicine to a more personalized and proactive approach is a necessity, the rehumanization of the system becomes necessary.

Human qualities such as sympathy, empathy, compassion, kindness, and healing touch have been for centuries the cornerstone of the art of medicine. With the incorporation of technology and artificial intelligence within the system in the near future, these human qualities are too valuable to be underestimated or discarded while making medicine more precise and cost-effective.

A renovated system needs to be built on four pillars—personalized care, proactive approach, human touch, and artificial intelligence—to deliver care in a more comprehensive way.

For medicine to continue providing care, and the system to regain people's trust and respect, priorities need to be reordered, with human emotions integrated into the main equation. Burnout is well-established as a public health problem within the healthcare profession, and suicides by physicians are increasing at an alarming rate. The technical progress and commercialization of healthcare have imposed new challenges, risking the lives of users and providers.

The public is wondering how people in caring professions can cease to care. Meanwhile, burnout, compassion fatigue, overwork, excess demands, lack of continuity, and new healthcare corporate efficiency markers and targets, such as early discharge, length of stay and readmission rates, make it harder for providers to treat patients as people. It's easy to lose the main thing that inspired them to become doctors in the first place—caring for and helping people.

An overemphasis on science overwhelms the need for understanding humanity. This may potentially grow even worse with the incorporation of artificial intelligence and more technology into the system, if it is done thoughtlessly.

A chasm has been created within the system, caused by a blame culture, punitive climate, and defensive practice. This has led to our profession traveling from one of the most rewarding to be seen now as one of the most liable and risky. Overcoming this, bridging or filling the chasm, will take a major restructuring of the current model. Efforts need to be redirected towards the human concepts of sympathy, empathy, compassion, kindness, and healing touch that I have summarized within the Four Pillars of Future Medicine.

Being tough and avoiding emotions to bring objectivity to the decision-making process has imposed an incalculable risk to the system, jeopardizing the sustainability of our profession. Depersonalization, existential neglect, and loss of human touch is alienating clinicians and patients. A culture that fosters competition rather than collaboration and an overemphasis on the evidence-based model of medicine are other factors threatening the continuity of the system itself, forcing more people to turn toward alternative options, such as chiropractors, naturopaths, and health coaches.

Human touch and hope have been proven to be instrumental for the healing process throughout history. As we learn more about how to optimize and collaborate with our own bodies' natural healing powers, it is imperative that we continue investing in efforts to better understand how emotions and human qualities impact these complex systems at all levels.

The body is in constant renewal. This renewal process depends on the quality of your stem cells and immune system. If stem and immune cells are healthy and well preserved, they can multiply more times and creating more new cells. As we age, stem and immune cells age with us, as we have discussed earlier. As stem and immune cells age, they lose their capacity to function, and they eventually degenerate and die. Studies have linked this process with the aforementioned deterioration of the biomolecular core, or microenvironment. The biomolecular harmony of the microenvironment depends on multiple factors. Micronutrient reserve, exosomes, stem cells, signaling nano-vesicles, toxins, and hormones all impact these complex processes, which explains why people heal at different paces and respond to health challenges differently.

Mounting evidence has proven that human touch, compassionate care, nurturing love, empathy, kindness, and healing touch all have the potential to activate healing mechanisms by changing the biomolecular harmony of the microenvironment: enhancing healing and tissue regeneration, slowing aging and preventing telomere shortening, aging-related functional decline, and chronic diseases.

As mentioned in page 111, UC Berkeley study was one of the first to demonstrate the effect of oxytocin, the love hormone, on stem cells. The researchers found that by giving oxytocin to old mice they were able to trigger muscle regrowth at a level comparable to young mice—far better than the old control group that didn't receive oxytocin. These results suggest that systemic administration of oxytocin may rapidly improve muscle healing and regeneration by enhancing aged muscle stem cell proliferation. This has lit up the field with hope, opening potential alternative mechanisms to explain how love and emotions impact our biology.

Love, compassion, and bonding are all connected to oxytocin, known as the "love or bonding hormone." Oxytocin is produced by both the provider and the receiver and brings benefits to both. An increasing number of studies suggest that compassionate care is linked to more patient and healthcare provider satisfaction. Studies also suggest that oxytocin enhances immune system function, wound healing, and may even kill cancer cells in vitro, while selectively helping immune cells to thrive. Although the role of oxytocin on all these beneficial effects is not completely understood, there is no question that the value of these elements is immeasurable.

Based on this science, I now recognize that the concept of love goes well beyond the romantic concept of being struck by Cupid's arrow or romantic love. Love, as postulated by Stefan Deutsch in his book *Love Decoded* and validated by Barbara Frederickson in her book, *Love 2.0*, is as essential as food, air, and water for humans to thrive. Today, it is broadly accepted that without nourishing love, children cannot grow and develop to their highest genetic potential. It is time to incorporate this concept of love into medicine, as it is obvious that nourishing love demonstrated through loving behaviors, such as compassion, empathy, and kindness are essential for human well-being, optimal thriving, personal development, and health. It is time for the concept of love to evolve from a philosophical discussion to a scientific fact. More studies need to be designed to solve the mystery of how love and the whole spectrum of loving behaviors, compassion, empathy, and kindness impact human health and development at the molecular level.

I dare to dream that one day, pushed by the efforts of leaders in the field of compassion and love, like Stefan Deutsch, Stephen Post, Barbara Frederickson, Jean Watson, Eva Selhub, and Matthieu Ricard, we would finally establish human touch and nourishing love as one of the foundational pillars of future medicine. Declaring our commitment to rehumanize medicine once and for all, we should guarantee that we never sacrifice the human factor again in our pursuit of a more effective, efficient, precise, and profitable system.

After all, nourishing love is essential to excel at a new health model that guarantees people a longer and better life. Our main purpose as healthcare leaders is to contribute to each individual's self-development, helping them become the best expression of themselves. This is something that has been neglected by our current system. And it should be fundamental to the concept of tomorrow's medicine.

No One Is YOU ... That Is Your Greatest Superpower

There is no greater superpower than the ability to discover, live, and embrace our most genuine and authentic self. No one is you and that is where your greatness lies. But we sometimes insist on adjusting ourselves to the environment, meeting loved ones' and others' expectations.

Being authentic means being the person you really want to be. That means letting go of anyone else's opinion of you, or their ideas about what you should be. It is about being present in the present moment, in the NOW, mindfully, with conviction, confidence, and awareness, staying true to yourself, letting go of expectations based on family traditions or cultural stereotypes. Embracing uncertainty fearlessly.

Aim to love your life and yourself unconditionally. Lose your facades—those multiple masks we decide to wear to prevent people from seeing who we really are. Embrace yourself. Embrace your process and who you are in the current moment and let go of your past and previous identities.

Going Naked

Up until yesterday,
I dressed my soul.
But today I get her out naked.
For brave? For reckless?
For crazy?
Or perhaps just for desperate...
'Cause who knows better than me,
that all the clothes of my prejudices
are weighing her down,
making our journey much harder.

Today, darling you're going out naked!
Today you will breathe without the weight of our own guilts,
and
you will feel the warmth of the sun and the refreshing summer breezes
without the boundaries self-imposed by our absurd shames.
Finally, awakening while learning what it means to really indulge in a hug,
a kiss,
a touch,
without either...
Fear or remorse,
past or future,
debts, or torments.

Today I witness a miracle!
Discovering how...
Joy transmutes to bliss,
silence transforms to celestial peace, and
love transcend the limitations of time and space
becoming infinite and divine.

> Today my soul is coming out naked, and
> I decide not to cover her anymore!

Ivel De Freitas, MD

Don't let fear of being rejected, judged, invalidated, financially crippled, or shamed stop you. Let your passion out. Give yourself permission to be, evolve, and grow.

Expectations are an illusion. We create them based on what we have learned it would be the ideal outcome. It is anticipating the future based on what it is acceptable and expected from you. Anticipating allows us to predict but leaves no room for surprises. Anticipating also disconnects you with your own life and reality, because life is not what should happen, but what is actually happening. I invite you to dream big, to let go your imagination, and move beyond your expectation. Writing your dreams with pen and your plan with pencil.

Although, I understand the concept of letting go expectation and embrace uncertainty may sound like I'm asking you to lower your bar. I invite you to explore the concept with an open mind, as your own expectation might become your own self-imposed limits. Instead, I want you to consider embracing the limitless spectrum of possibilities embedded in the ocean of uncertainty.

Just by embracing uncertainty you can connect with the now opening new gates, removing limiting belief and setting you free to recognize opportunities and accomplish what you want on your own terms and develop your talents as superpowers.

By understanding that everyone has a special set of abilities that any of us may potentially unfold by aligning self-unique talents, with purpose, discipline, and love, it is what has driven me to contemplate the possibility of collaborating in the recreation of a new model for healthcare. A model that focuses on helping each individual to upgrade his/her/they biology, unleash his/her/their genetic potential and become the absolute best version of his/her/they-self.

As higher consciousness is the next stage of human evolution and progress is reaching an exponential growth phase, we need to rise, and the best way to do it is embracing and honoring key concepts such as inclusiveness, diversity, and bioindividuality. It is about time for us to understand that we are all special in our own way and that our differences are meant to make us stronger. A philosophy that has become more rooted to my soul and that I have laid out in many of my poems, especially on "Welcome to a New World" published at the beginning of this book.

I am convinced that these concepts are key to aging *beyond well*. Aging should be a process of accomplishment and celebration, as the person you are becoming is always better than the person you have been. I like me today more than me ten years ago, but I like more the person I am becoming: a more authentic, beautiful, spiritual, sophisticated—with a little hint of irreverence, wiser, fitter, healthier, and happier human. I am definitively becoming a better version of me. So, although I know my skin will not ever be the same, I could care less. As I mentioned in the introduction of this book, don't fear aging, be scared of stagnation, dullness, and spiritual idleness. After all, our legacy will be our consciousness.

Artificial Intelligence Is Here to Stay

There is no question that artificial intelligence (AI) is key to moving healthcare and medicine to the next level and one of the pillars for future medicine. With the incorporation of the genome into everyone's profile, the need for a more advanced technology that allows us to use this extensive and complex data to benefit the individual patient is imperative. The traditional medicine model assigns drugs or treatment based on the needs of the statistically average person with a particular diagnosis. Disruptive technologies that incorporate more complex data into our current algorithms need to be embraced and implemented. Microchips carrying your genome sequence as part of your picture ID, and AI are technological advancements that seem to be the solution to the challenge.

As disruptive technologies keep materializing on the stage of healthcare, it becomes possible to get down even more deeply to the roots of diseases and create personalized strategies based on bioindividuality, or even beyond that—the Bioindividuality 2.0 model, which means made and tailored just for you and not for people like you.

> "Exponential growth is seductive, starting out slowly and virtually unnoticeably, but beyond the knee of the curve it turns explosive and profoundly transformative. The future is widely

misunderstood. Our forebears expected to be pretty much like their present, which had been pretty much like their past. Exponential trends did exist a thousand years ago, but they were at that very early stage in which they were so flat and so slow that they looked like there were not trend at all. As a result, observers' expectations of an unchanged future was fulfilled."

—Ray Kurzweil from *Singularity is Near*

With the incorporation of more disruptive technologies, such as AI, into healthcare, the traditional approach of "one-size-fits-all" will definitely start to crumble. Currently, we know that everyone has a different genetic code, may react differently to pharmaceuticals, or may have a completely opposite reaction to treatment than assumed. So why should we treat everyone with the same drugs or with the same method? To be able to understand individual variability in genes, environment, and lifestyle for each person, medicine must embrace more efficient software and AI engines that allow doctors to gather, analyze, and store incredible amounts of information.

This huge need for limitless data analytics is one area where AI comes into the medical arena. Within a couple of years, it will be the only way to analyze the amount of medical data for each individual, find new correlations based on existing precedents, and draw accurate and reliable conclusions. It will become the doctor-patient's best support in decision-making.

It raises the question: If the AI engine analyzes the data and tells us what to do, what will the doctor's job be? Which is where human touch becomes even more important for us to develop and understand.

I have no doubts that AI will be the stethoscope of the twenty-first century and the backbone of personalized medicine. We are not there yet, and there is a lot of debate on the safety and liability of bringing AI into medicine. But we must start preparing for what is definitely coming in the near future. A big part of this preparation is better understanding the power of human touch at the center of medicine and averting the possibility of AI becoming an existential threat to humankind as feared by some people.

At least I think it never will. As I said before, the art of medicine comprises a deep understanding of human emotions, not just gathering symptoms and assigning a diagnosis. Human qualities such as empathy, compassion, and kindness are too complex and too valuable to be discarded when incorporating AI. After all, these human qualities are the main components of the art of medicine, and authentic and genuine art should remain a human quality despite progress.

Andrew McAfee, a leader at the MIT Sloan School of Management Center for Digital Business, in one of the videos from Big Think, brilliantly discussed the question of AI replacing human qualities, such as creativity. He states that AIs can create original "works of art" and follow any protocol even more accurately than the highest-skilled human being, if they receive some guidance. But they certainly don't have any awareness of the fundamental conditions of being human, such as being aware of our own mortality, living inside a designated physical body, and, most importantly, interacting with and relating to other humans.

Based on a strict definition of creativity as the ability to produce something novel and valuable, AI technically could qualify as creative. Luckily for us humans, though, experts don't think AI will ever be able to understand the human condition and emotions with the depth and complexity of a human brain. We seem to be very far from a point where algorithms would allow AI to practice genuine empathy and compassion, reflecting our emotions back and meeting our needs in a meaningful and transcendental way.

> "I'm skeptical we're going to be able to successfully convey that intuition even to a really big, really sophisticated piece of technology. If that day ever comes, it's a long way away."
>
> **—Andrew McAfee**

If this best-case scenario proves true, it becomes imperative to shift our personal development goals toward developing more emotional, spiritual, and even erotic intelligence. Areas in which we cannot be yet replaced or surpassed so as to prevent rendering ourselves obsolete. Also, this prevents us from relinquishing the final quality that differentiates us from machines and makes us human: love, compassion, creativity, spirituality, and sexuality.

Ray Kurzweil, who predicts immortality for 2045, describes these changes as the next step in our evolution. In a *Playboy* interview, Kurzweil said, "We'll create more profound forms of communication than we're familiar with today, more profound music and funnier jokes. We'll be funnier. We'll be sexier. We'll be more adept at expressing loving sentiments."

We'll be more emotionally intelligent. Don't you like that in our future?

We Are in Fact Getting There

Although it seems we still have a long way to go, it is time to get started! It is our responsibility to build the foundation and prepare for what is coming. The way to start is by challenging the status quo and believing that your health and spiritual development are as important as your professional, financial, and academic development. How machines are going to surpass us in the near future should inspire changes in education, healthcare, and business at the legislation and regulation levels but also at your own personal development level.

Some of those changes are already happening. We see it in the way our approach to certain challenges has changed. But we can't stop. Evolution and challenge need to be the steppingstones of our daily living, perceiving it as an opportunity instead of an obstacle.

How I have done that in my personal life and practice is how I approach fatigue and burnout. These conditions are associated with the wear and tear of chronic stress on your biomolecular core. They are widely recognized as manifestations of specific micronutrient deficiencies. However, the reactive character of traditional blood tests and the lack of a gold standard to exactly measure your biomolecular core has prevented doctors and scientists from being more proactive and recognizing the importance of this biomolecular gap. I decided a long time ago to take this as an opportunity to explore new technologies to find better ways to treat these common conditions.

By harnessing cutting-edge biomolecular and genomic technology, our team has been able to create an innovative health system that gets to the core of your health, identifies what is missing, and formulates a personalized formula to fix it.

Our formula originally combined only micronutrients. We are in the process of incorporating peptides and stem cell–based bioactive products, better known as exosomes, into our research protocols. The goal is to find innovative, proactive, and personalized methods to upgrade health and life by optimizing and harmonizing the individual biomolecular core. Growing evidence suggests this may boost an individual's immune system and the capacity of stem cells to regenerate naturally, slowing down their aging process.

Thankfully, we are not alone. Many other groups with similar visions are working hard to make things change. Yet, the majority of physicians in the field of functional medicine are working with protocols designed to treat a condition or medical problem: fatigue, eczema, headaches, adrenal fatigue, migraines, dry skin, Parkinson's, autoimmune disorders, and so on, following a traditional diagnosis-centered approach. There are other groups working toward making medicine more sensitive to this biomolecular individuality. Individuals like Deepak Chopra, Mark Hyman, James Lavalle, Pam Smith, Andrew Heyman, Naveen Jain, and many others, whose inspiring influences and contributions are making possible the shift in status quo that is needed to foster the open-minded and innovative environment that is so needed to move to our next milestone. They all understand that with the development in the last few years of new diagnostics, genomics, and information technology the doors opened to the possibility of providing a more tailored and targeted approach.

My vision is that the foundation of your health, quality of life, and longevity lies in the biomolecular core. To continue moving medicine to a more proactive and patient-centered approach, we need to embrace this system. This means we need to focus our efforts on creating a better understanding of the needs of this core. Understanding that the missing pieces of this core compromise the trillion biochemical processes that determine not only how fast you age, how well your immune system protects you, and how well your genes express, but also how good you look, act, and feel in your everyday life.

It might take many years before we see this approach become standard of care and for insurance companies to evolve to support more proactive approach. But I hope you realize that gaining access to this advancement is open today for those willing to be part of it and contribute to this promising field.

Imagine what medicine would be if whenever you came to the doctor for your regular checkup you were infused with a formula to optimize your internal processes and upgrade your biology. Imagine your inner chemistry being reset from survival/inflammatory/aging to healing/recovery/rejuvenating mode. Imagine turning *on* and *off* certain genes to help you unleash your greatest genetic potentials.

Therefore, whenever you get sick and come to the hospital for attention, before they give you anything, they will have infused you with your personal upgrading formula to power up your immune system and enhance your natural healing powers. Wouldn't this be the best way to get well? This could decrease the need for medication and hospitalizations. I have my own practice to prove it. I have done that. I have been there. This is one of the reasons I came out of the closet and wrote this book. I know sincerely that we are ready. As Ray Kurzweil said: "Inventing is a lot like surfing: you have to anticipate and catch the wave at just the right moment."

I know we are there.

By understanding what your core is missing we are acting before the deficiency creates a problem. It allows us to create a strategy and a specific formula to fix the deficiency, preventing the problem from developing. Don't you think this is common sense and should be taken to create the foundation of a real proactive approach? Can you imagine remodeling our current healthcare model to match this vision? An approach that can be used regardless of age, gender, race, medical history, or health status. An approach that targets real prevention and cure from the biomolecular core out, instead of early diagnosis and disease management. An approach that brings in real-time tangible improvement in the areas of life that really matters to *you*: energy, vitality, brain clarity, gut health, sleep, mood, peace of mind, sex drive, skin, nails, and hair.

Joining Efforts

As the regulatory environment becomes more complex, the costs for the small compounding pharmacies to manufacture personalized products becomes unsustainable. Many of these pharmacies have disappeared, and the ones that have managed to survive are struggling. To continue they need to produce more and in bulk, making the concept of personalization even more challenging. I have been working with different compounding pharmacies over the last few years, and some of them have closed their doors while others have stopped producing sterile products to stay in business.

I am not saying that regulations are unnecessary. However, everything from standard of care to research and technology are built on and in support of the diagnosis-centered, pharma-lobbying, and reactive medical model that is becoming more corporative and less humanistic as we speak. Meaning that regulations are based on sustaining this model, preventing the advancement of a more patient-centered and proactive approach.

The lack of scientific consensus and lack of economic interest have eclipsed the development of this field and affected the sustainability of compounding pharmacies. I work only with pharmacies that go beyond meeting standards. I visit them personally and support them as much as I can. I have put together a board of experts in my effort to try to preserve the compounding pharmacy and other labs in the industry. But as you can imagine this is not easy. This requires creating a network of pharmacies and physicians and developing a consensus on marketing/education strategies to ensure that the public learns more about this challenge, at least this is my vision.

I must admit that I have been very fortunate, as my efforts have not gone completely unnoticed. From Silicon Valley to international software development corporations and research institutions, my ideas have been heard and supported. We are currently creating a platform to translate these progressive therapeutic methods into advanced algorithms that I envision will help us to create a database that can support the progress of this field. I know it sounds huge and ambitious. But since I have made it my mission to recreate biomolecular therapy to rethink and reshape medicine, I cannot moderate and limit my vision. This is me dreaming big. I hope that my efforts can contribute to the work of others who share the same vision of "healthy longevity and life of fulfillment for all"—meaning the roughly eight billion people of the world.

CHAPTER 11

The Best Is Yet to Come

Cellular health enhancement, genetic expression regulation, telomere elongation, lifespan prolongation and targeted tissue rejuvenation and regeneration are among the many benefits that can be safely achieved by translating to practice the complex scientific evidence available today.

We know that the foundation of your health, quality of life and longevity lies in your biomolecular core, composed of your own biochemical and genetic makeup. Missing pieces of this core, combined with aging and proinflammatory signals from your own cells, can compromise the delicate harmony of the trillion biochemical processes that determine not only how fast you age but also how well you look, act, and feel.

By harnessing cutting-edge biomolecular and genomic technology, we have created an innovative health system that can get to the core of your health. By providing a better understanding of what you are missing, you create your own formula aiming to fix it.

Our formula combines micronutrients and antioxidants initially, then adds peptides and stem cell bioactive products, better known as exosomes, as our research project aims to enhance the scope of these innovative anti-aging therapeutic protocols. The goal is to upgrade individual health and life by optimizing individual biomolecular core harmony, which accumulating evidence suggests may naturally boost immune and stem cell regenerative capacities.

While the use of technology is key to the biohacking movement, the main goal is to understand how we can really make technology help us live longer, healthier, and happier lives. One great example are the biological age calculators, like our *Immunity Age Calculator* designed to help you track your immune system's age. This is a term we use to define what age your immune system "acts" like, which may reflect how good your immune response can potentially be not only when fighting infection, but also responding to vaccination. Just because you are a certain age, doesn't mean your body and immune system will respond the same way as most people in your age group. During COVID-19 we learned that *aging healthily* seems to be one of the most protective factors for complications and mortality. It is not so much your chronological age that actually predicts your risk of complications, but perhaps your immunity age. We are also learning that our immune system is key regulating the aging signals and the ticking of our body's clock. So, learning and monitoring your immunity age becomes very important to understand the aging pace of your overall body and choose the right lifestyle strategies to potentially slow down your clock. Although technology sounds complicated for some people, on the quest to stay healthy, technology can give us an edge in our personal and professional lives. I invite you to check your immunity age for free in our website: www.onogen.com and check your Epigenetic DNA Age which reports your Immunity DNA Age as well with the in-home TruAge kit testing that you can get at www.trudiagnostic.com or on our website or any of our offices (by the way I have no financial connection with Trudiagnostic).

Biohacking Immunity to Redefine Aging

As the field of multi-omic diagnostic and therapeutics evolve, we are doing our part to further the use of epigenetic methylation testing in clinical application.

While the pandemic is waking up the world to a global immune reset and a change in healthcare, we are developing a study, designed to test an innovative biohacking medical model, combining the latest of science and technology to deliver personalized medicine safely.

I want to add that this protocol was shared with different people connected with the Florida and New York Departments of Health at the beginning of the pandemic. I also gathered different leaders of the field. Together I was envisioning we could create a stronger effect collaborating in the creation of better protocols to face the threat imposed by the pandemic. Although our efforts were ignored, data published from abroad support the beneficial effects that all these proposed therapies, including the controversial use of thymosin alpha 1. As I have mentioned, anything that helps your body preserve and modulate your immunity should have a protective effect until proven otherwise.

To facilitate the delivery and implementation of our program we have developed a three-phase protocol aimed at upgrading an individual's biology, resetting inner chemistry to healing mode, and biohacking some of your natural healing genetic powers.

The program is designed to be delivered under an Institutional Review Board (IRB) clinical trial. IRB is a group that has been formally designated to review and monitor biomedical research involving human research. This group review serves an important role in the protection of the rights and welfare of human research subjects. We are currently recruiting patients who are interested in participating.

The trial is designed to not only deliver your personalized anti-aging and immunity optimization plan on-demand to you, from the comfort of your own house or office, but it also takes less than thirty minutes per visit and requires just a few visits a year.

The whole model is designed to guarantee scalability, aiming to collaborate on the process of creating a new biomolecular and more proactive medical foundation to help in the process of rethinking and reshaping the healthcare system moving forward.

Personalized recommendations are all generated after filling out a comprehensive biohacking medical questionnaire and a comprehensive biomolecular profiling that includes determination of an individual's Immunity DNA Age. The prototype is already available in our website: www.onogen.com. The protocols are assigned based on proprietary therapeutic algorithms designed to specifically address those biomolecular gaps and imbalances even before they manifest as symptoms and/or medical problems.

This trial is also aiming to validate a pioneering software platform, envisioned to become the foundation to the first AI Medical Engine designed to deliver Personalized Biomolecular Medicine Protocols with the main goal to create a new, precise, personalized, proactive, empowering, inclusive, and patient-centered medical model to disrupt and renovate the one in place.

Individual protocols will all be comprised of three different phases that might be delivered all during the first therapy or in different therapeutic sessions depending upon an individual's medical profiling:

PRIME

ONOGEN PRIME, the phase I of ONOGEN biohacking medical protocol, is designed to provide patients with our signature physician selection of specific biomolecular active ingredients – micronutrients, minerals, methyl factors and antioxidants.

Founded on the belief that we operate most of the time at just a fraction of our full potential due to unrecognized gaps within our biomolecular and nutritional core. This approach intends to upgrade your biology nutritionally, to support your body, genes, and mind to achieve their full biomolecular and genetic potential.

Each patient's personalized PRIME formula will be specifically designed to meet individual's unique biomolecular cellular needs and optimize DNA methylation which has been found to greatly impact genes' health, promoting good genes to express better and preventing bad genes turning on. These therapies are all personalized for each patient based on the results of their online medical assessment and the results of cutting-edge biomolecular lab testing.

Each patient's PRIME protocol may consist of one or multiple sessions depending on their personal biomolecular needs. Other oral enhancers or testing may be added to each personalized plan to address further possible deficiencies.

RESET

RESET, the phase II of the protocol, is specifically designed to switch the body's inner chemistry from inflammation/aging mode to healing/anti-aging mode.

Founded on the belief that the body's inner chemistry is in constant motion, switching from survival/stress mode to healing/recovering mode allows the body to keep that delicate balance needed for the body to recover and heal optimally, slowing down aging.

As we mentioned previously in the first part of this book, this balance depends upon a delicate signaling system produced by your own stem cells and immune system, known as exosomes. Filled with healing messages, these nano-sized communication vesicles decrease inflammation and prevent immunosenescence.

By combining cutting-edge neuroimmune behavioral strategies—such as meditation, biofeedback, and practices that enhance loving inner chemistry—with the novel science of exosomes, once your body has been primed, this phase is targeted to enhance patient's natural coping, healing, and recovery powers, aiming to help the body to become more resilient, cope with stress better, age less, and achieve more in the day-to-day with less effort.

Still under investigation, exosomes' potent anti-inflammatory and immunomodulating natural effects have become a promising nanomedicine clinical tool for the treatment and prevention of different aging and age-related diseases. At present, therapeutic use of exosomes is still under research.

GO

GO, protocol phase III, is specifically designed to enhance body's natural healing and rejuvenation powers by naturally enhancing specific genes' expression.

Based on the science of peptides, short fragments of amino acids, normally produced by the body, this phase is founded on the belief that body's natural healing and recovery powers can be enhanced.

Peptides produced replicating the ones naturally produced by the body have been found to be key to repair tissue and even gene's alterations that may occur with aging, stress, and chronic inflammation.

Our body is meant to heal and stay healthy. Still under investigation, peptides' specific genetic activation powers are one of the most promising therapeutic tools under development and investigation today.

Creating Tomorrow's Medicine Today!

The pandemic has come to bring us a new insight to the key role *immune resilience* and immunosenescense, the natural decline of your immunity with aging, plays not only for defining your chance of overcoming COVID-19 successfully but also defining and pacing your own individual aging process and quality of life.

The younger we are, the easier we overcome colds and simple bacterial infections. The older we get the less resilient our body and immune system become.

However, even young people are now experiencing the same immune-declining phenomenon, although in their case is not related to age but to their stress perception level. The more stress you feel the less resilient your immune system may become. Our immune system is meant to balance itself, but as our immune system ages or it's marinated in the inner chemistry of survival and stress mode, we all seem to experience a progressive reduction of our immune system resilience. As we all collectively lose our immune resilience, growing amounts of evidence and demographic data suggest that we might be accelerating the process of biological aging at a molecular level, triggering and worsening many aging-related chronic conditions, such as dementia, arthritis, heart disease, and cancer, which is exactly what our demographics are showing and continue predicting.

One of the main lessons we should all learn from this pandemic is to not take our immune system for granted. Taking vitamin C, vitamin D, and zinc has become a new norm to keep immunity strong and stay healthy, demonstrating some level of collective awakening towards this subject. More doctors and scientists, like myself, are looking into better and safe innovative ways to build immune resilience to prevent getting infected in the first place, help people develop a robust long-lasting immunity after the infection or vaccination, and prevent lung injury and other complications that increase mortality in those who acquire COVID-19. But why do some people become extremely ill, but not others? Why do symptoms vary so drastically among patients? How can we build immune resilience and defeat aging?

As well as endeavoring to answer these questions, we believe that identifying and decoding the signals emitted by our immune systems could be key to enabling improved not only COVID-19 patient management, but also adding a new biomolecular approach to to slow down the fundamental aging process and lessen its impact.

If all this sound interesting to you I invite to sign up in our website for a chance to participate in a biohacking experience. Participants will be provided medical therapies and data on the following:

- Biological and Immunity Epigenetic DNA Age
- Telomeres
- Immune Health
- Inflammation
- Pace of Aging
- Longevity

This pioneering study aims to explore novel diagnostic and therapeutic insights to give individuals immunity enhancement and healthy longevity and find ways to bring it to the general public.

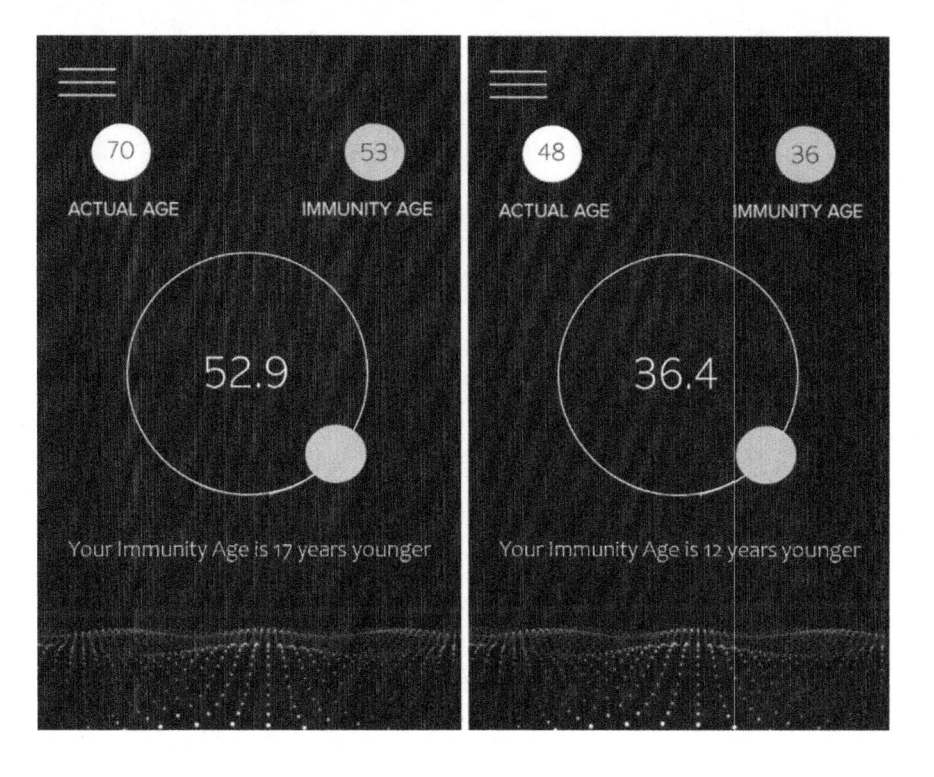

ACTUAL AGE	IMMUNITY AGE	ACTUAL AGE	IMMUNITY AGE
70	53	48	36
52.9		36.4	
Your Immunity Age is 17 years younger		Your Immunity Age is 12 years younger	

230 | Aging Beyond Well

ACTUAL AGE	IMMUNITY AGE	ACTUAL AGE	IMMUNITY AGE
48	27	52	43

26.9
Your Immunity Age is 21 years younger

43.2
Your Immunity Age is 9 years younger

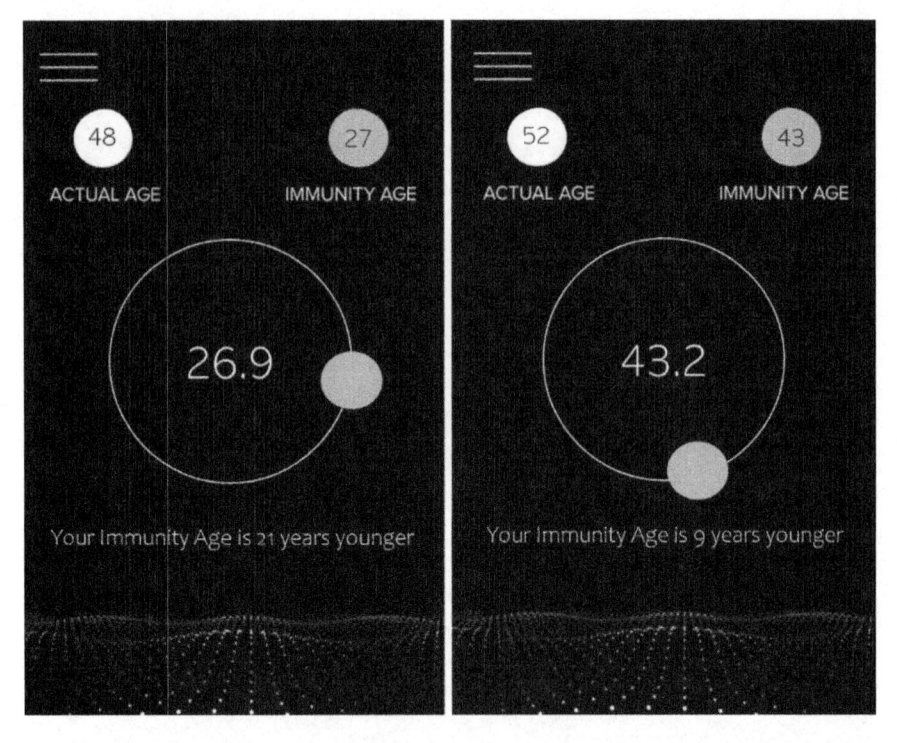

Our preliminary results show a mean improvement of an individual's Immunity Epigenetic DNA Age and telomere DNA length increasing up to 35 percent when patients follow our initial protocols for a year. Here are a few examples of our patients' results: the first one is 70 years old but her immunity age is 52.9; the second one is 48 years old and her immunity age is 36.4; the third one is 48 and her immunity age is 26; and the fourth one is 52 and his immunity age is 43.

We envision this becoming a movement that help to expedite the breaking of the old paradigms and redefining a new model that champions patient preference, intuition, and values as equal to medical expertise.

What's Next?

Just imagine what is next—engineered exosomes to deliver specific peptides, missing factors, or healing signals to specific cells and tissues and immune cells engineered to kill specific viruses or cancer cells without harming other cells, just like the advancements we are all seeing with, NK

(Natural Killer Cells) universal vaccines, and CAR-T cells. CAR-T cell therapy is a form of immunotherapy that uses specially altered immune cells to fight cancer.

We now know that age, chronic diseases, environmental factors, and genetic characteristics can all interfere with how our stem cells communicate with other cells, thus disrupting the healing process through their gene expression. Today we are capable of overcoming those challenges by isolating exosomes from stem cell cultures or from fluid rich in exosomes, such as amniotic fluid and activating particular genes using specific peptides.

Exosomes and peptides are, in my opinion, two of the most promising and exciting therapeutic tools on the horizon. They are being heralded as the new frontier of acellular regenerative therapies because they play a vital role in the communication, modulation, and rejuvenation of all cells in our body, without the downside of using cells.

Increasing evidence is demonstrating that the positive effects of stem cell therapy, mostly derived from bone marrow, adipose tissue, and perinatal products, are greatly mediated by exosomes. The signals released from the mediated cells and not the stem cells themselves are the main factors that activate the patient's own cells to heal and regenerate.

The question now is, do we skip the cells and give patients exosomes and get the same effect?

Early evidence suggests that this could be the case, and exosomes could displace cell therapy. Promising results have been seen using exosomes in patients with stroke, lost neurological function, skin wounds, and chronic conditions, as well as patient with acute lung injury related to COVID-19 and patients with post COVID syndrome. There is also evidence of accelerated healing, new skin formation, and improved functionality in degenerative arthritis that keeps patients from requiring surgery broadly documented in the literature.

Peptides, on the other hand, are short fragments of amino acids, normally produced by your body, which have been found to be the key to repair tissue and even modulate immunity and gene alterations that may occur with aging, stress, and chronic inflammation.

Peptides are naturally found in your body, they are very potent, highly selective, and do not produce toxic metabolites. They are used to create extremely specific reactions in your body.

Peptides are different from hormones, as they are smaller molecules that stimulate your own body production of certain hormones and healing factors.

While hormones are essential for the balance of many of your body's key functions, peptides' unique mechanism brings the benefits of preventing the undesired effect of hormone production shutting down, often seen with hormone replacement. There has been evidence of enhanced immunity against viruses and some kind of cancers, accelerated healing of wounds and ligament tears, and improved functionality in degenerative arthritis with the use of different peptides.

But what's next? Can we identify what particular factors and peptides patients are missing and proactively add them to a formula we can administer periodically to ensure patient's cells communicate optimally and tissues heal and regenerate better? Could we enhance the healing effect of other therapeutic approaches by understanding an individual's weaknesses and provide the factors needed to overcome them? The science to get to this level exists in progress. Although still unavailable for widespread commercial use, I have no doubt that it will soon become available, as has happened with genetic testing that has hit the market in recent years. To you it may feel as if there is no rush, yet I know people who are eagerly expecting these changes to happen sooner than later so they can significantly improve their quality of life.

Good examples are Pricilla and Mark. They are two of my patients who underwent adipose-derived stem cell treatment after biomolecular optimization. Despite their presumed diagnosis of secondary progressive multiple sclerosis, a disease in which the immune system eats away at the protective covering of nerves, they both experienced some improvements.

In MS, resulting nerve damage disrupts communication between the brain and the body. MS causes many different symptoms, including vision loss, pain, fatigue, and impaired coordination and gait. The symptoms, severity, and duration can vary from person to person. Some people may be symptom-free most of their lives, while others may have symptoms that come and go in frequent crises, or linger, causing severe neurological impairment and disability that never go away.

In their case, they both had gait impairment, requiring walking with a rolling walker. Mark was in his early forties and Pricilla was in her early fifties. They both described heat intolerance, fatigue, urinary frequency, and urgency, which they said was very disruptive for their day-to-day routine. Pricilla loves to travel to the Caribbean islands, but as the disease progressed her heat intolerance and urinary frequency made these trips harder and more challenging. Mark loves to watch his kids' sports events, but the same symptoms prevented him from being outside too long. Both patients hated the idea of taking immunosuppressants to control the disease, because the extensive list of side effects and risk of adverse reactions seemed to be as bad as the disease itself.

After they were treated with our protocol of biomolecular optimization followed by an infusion of their own adipose-derived stem cells, they both experienced improvement of their quality of life, and disease progression, fatigue, heat intolerance, and urinary symptoms improved radically. Although gait impairment and neurological deficit did not reverse for them as I have described in other patients with previous strokes or TBI, they both recognized that their quality of life improved significantly after the therapy, and their disease progression seemed to slow down.

But why weren't stem cells able to help them to recover from their neurological damage? Why did they help people with strokes but not these people with MS?

Here's the most possible answer of why: We now know that inflammation plays an important role in the brain damage process that follows a stroke. Although many aspects of local inflammation at the stroke site are beneficial and aimed at restoring tissue balance, collateral damage by the acute inflammatory response plays an important role in the persistence of neurological deficit. While many aspects of inflammation are beneficial and aimed at restoring brain tissue balance, collateral damage by the acute inflammatory response contributes to ischemic damage. As I mentioned before, there is strong evidence that most of the immune modulation and anti-inflammatory effects attributed to stem cells are due to exosomes. Exosomes may play a functional role in regulating the adaptive immune response after a stroke or in autoimmune disease and limit the negative effect of post-stroke inflammation.

This immune-modulatory response may explain the effect seen in Mark and Pricilla, as their disease stopped progressing, and some symptoms were resolved. However, the therapy was not able to rebuild the damaged nerves. Despite the therapy may have created a modulatory effect on the immune system, the kind of reset that allows the immune system to stop or decrease fighting its own tissue, the therapy was probably not able to turn on mechanisms that rebuild nerves. This is one of the areas I think engineered exosomes loaded with specific nerve growth factors and genetic signals would be needed to be able to overcome those therapeutic challenges.

In the meantime, significant numbers of patients who have been treated as part of the multiple IRB Research Projects in progress in the country with cell-therapy or exosomes are reporting a generalized rejuvenating effect in preliminary reports. This makes us think they could be a potential ally in the development of the youth elixir we are all dreaming for.

Based on my observations and research, the perfect combination for such a formula is micronutrients, peptides, and exosomes. Although, based on my clinical observation and research, with today's technology and algorithms that I have been developing, I feel I am getting closer to being able to personalize the micronutrients and some peptides based on Bioindividuality 2.0, and the exosomes based on advanced inflammatory markers efficiently for patients. I cannot wait for the level of technology that will allow us to bring an even more advanced level of bioindividuality to our protocols. By that I mean, we would start using engineered exosomes with the specific genetic information and growth factors that you were missing to help you achieve your highest potential, not only in terms of longevity and quality of life, but in self-development and expression of individual talents.

The Elixir of Youth: Is This Really Possible?

Looking for this elixir of youth formula has been in the minds of scientists and visionaries for centuries. In the 1950s, researchers connected the circulatory systems of old mice to young mice to determine its effects. They found that the old mice experienced numerous rejuvenating effects. Many biomarkers of youth returned, and the mice lived longer. The younger mice connected to older mice also had shorter lifespans.

Parabiosis experiments died out in the 1970s, partly because researchers had learned what they could from the technique, and regulations on animal research, thankfully, have made it more challenging to conduct this kind of experiments, protecting animals from experimentation and cruel practices. However, the data obtained has helped us to learn more about the importance of aging signaling. Today we recognize that a significant part of the rejuvenating effect seen in the old mice and the aging effect seen in the young mice were likely mediated by exosomes. Evidence is pointing at exosomes as great mediators in the aging response, because while cells are young, with long telomeres, they produce exosomes richer in growth and healing factors. But as cells are damaged and telomeres get shorter, exosomes become more like self-destructive signals than regenerating signals. This explains why the young mice's lifespan shortened by being connected with the old mice.

Evidence also suggests that love may have been playing a role in this rejuvenating effect seen in the parabiosis research. Higher levels of oxytocin were observed in the young mice's blood compared to the old peers. As we have explained before, oxytocin has been linked to regeneration and cellular growth. Therefore, exosomes and oxytocin may explain part of the rejuvenating effect because they both are capable of activating stem cells throughout the body, helping to heal damage, replace cells and increase organ function.

So, love and exosomes, nutrients and peptides seem to be the key ingredients for an ideal Elixir of Youth, and efforts should be directed towards them.

It is clear, that although we are still in the preliminary research stage, we are developing a better understanding of how our biomolecular core and cellular microenvironment are essential for health, quality of life, and healthy longevity. There is also enough evidence to believe that emotions and thoughts exert their impact by influencing the microenvironment and biomolecular core, explaining in part why stress and a broken heart can precipitate changes in our genes as much as love and fulfillment.

In order to truly answer these questions and bring the field into the mainstream, we need to responsibly call out all those who are abusing or jeopardizing this promising field and help to redesign the system to become more flexible, but still within a safe and regulated environment.

Clinical trials will need to evolve. In *Nature*, "Personalized medicine: Time for one-person trial," Nicholas Schork stated, "Precision medicine requires a different type of clinical trial that focuses on individual, not average, responses to therapy." Research protocols need to be recreated to take into consideration bioindividuality, and software needs to be designed to support this complex target. The grant assignment and data collection process need to become a more friendly and collective process that allows better control and more automatic database collection.

In the meantime, I really hope that the knowledge and advice I have shared with you in this book can help you to achieve enhanced, upgraded well-being, empowering you to become one of those privileged individuals who gets to walk and enjoy the pathway beyond standard, to being *beyond well*.

Please remember that science, as it is now, is not enough. In order to get there, you need to combine it with love and spirituality. Self-acceptance, self-compassion and kindness are as important in this process as perseverance, determination, and discipline. The final goal is to become the best, truest and highest version of yourself every day. Yes, the goal is to become every day a healthier, happier, funnier, smarter, and sexier version of *you*.

Embrace your look at every age. Stay focused on the here and now—not what you looked like twenty years ago—it's key. Nothing is sexier than self-acceptance, loving embodiment, and authenticity. Focus on your energy, on your gains, on who you are becoming.

Embrace your process with the eyes of an explorer, the soul of a child, the flexibility of a contortionist, the tenacity of a marathonist, that adaptability of a salamander, and the enthusiasm of a new lover.

Keep changing. Keep asking. Keep growing. Keep evolving. Keep succeeding. Keep moving. Keep shining…

Learn to let go and laugh. Stay lighthearted. Stay intact. Be a kid. Laugh at yourself. Be kind, forgive and love, love, love yourself, passionately and unconditionally. Flirt with your potentials. Romance with your dreams. Acknowledge and stretch your ego. Get engaged with simplicity and authenticity. Be married your truest self.

As Picasso once said, "it takes a long time to become young." I would add and a lot of courage, spiritual self-work and growth, stretching the ego, and building up the muscles of patience and unconditional self-love.

Remember, aging should be a process of accomplishment and celebration, because the person you are becoming is always better than the person you've been. Don't be afraid of aging; be afraid of stagnation, dullness, and spiritual idleness. Learn to trust yourself and the power of love! In the pure frequency of love lies the secret path for oneness. Love is all; all is you. *Love* vibrates at an extremely high frequency of *energy*. Love is endless, love transcends. Love is the force that can make us immortal.

Love is All. All is You!

Love,
one person's muse,
another person's grief.
Vital energy!
Essential requirement
to achieve true happiness.

Mythified, vilified, manipulated,
distorted, mistreated, misused, and
even abused.
Tenacious, intrepid, and audacious,
It firmly stands by,
in humble understanding of its
crucial role as vital force.
Patiently waiting for us
to finally awaken,
understand and accept
the only way to love is
unconditionally.

Unconditional love,
without sense of ownership,
but with sense of belonging.
Belonging to the feeling,
to that vital energy
that's generated only by love.
Belonging that generates security.
Security that no matter what happens
love will never end!

Love beyond actions and words.
Love beyond time and events.
Love that survives any challenge.
Love that never dies,
but grows, transforms,
enhances.

Love to cultivate.
Love to transmute
to that better version of our vulnerable humanity that waits for us confidently.
I hope we have the courage to arrive and surrender to its sacred vital force!
Perhaps that's heaven?
Perhaps immortality?
Perhaps...

Ivel De Freitas, MD

What does aging mean for you? Let's start changing the concept.

Namaste—the light in me loves and honors the light in you.

Printed in Great Britain
by Amazon